TABLE OF CONTENTS

PREFACE   2

CHAPTER1: SYSTEMATIC REVIEW AND META-ANALYSIS: AN OVERVIEW WITH THE HELP OF R SOFTWARE   3

CHAPTER2: STRUCTURAL EQUATION MODELLING IN THE BIOMEDICAL DOMAIN: CONCEPTS AND METHODS REVISITED WITH THE HELP OF R STATISTICAL PACKAGE   17

CHAPTER3: AN OVERVIEW OF CLINICAL TRIAL DATA MANAGEMENT, ITS STANDARDS AND RECENT TRENDS   29

CHAPTER4: NATURAL LANGUAGE PROCESSING CONCEPTS AND METHODS REVISITED   39

CHAPTER5: FACTOR ANALYSIS REVISITED – AN OVERVIEW WITH THE HELP OF SPSS, SAS AND R PACKAGES   48

CHAPTER6: POST-HOC AND MULTIPLE COMPARISON TEST – AN OVERVIEW WITH SAS AND R STATISTICAL PACKAGE   65

CHAPTER7: APPLICATION OF QUANTILE REGRESSION IN CLINICAL RESEARCH: AN OVERVIEW WITH THE HELP OF R AND SAS STATISTICAL PACKAGE   78

PREFACE

This book is an edited book from the papers of International Journal of Statistics and Medical Informatics (IJSMI) authored by Editor, International of Journal of Statistics and Medical Informatics. It covers topics such as systematic review and meta-analysis, factor analysis, structural equation modelling and quantile regression in the field of biomedical domain. It also provides insight into the post hoc comparison, clinical trail data management and natural language processing methods.

Editor
International Journal of Statistics and Medical Informatics (IJSMI)

Chapter1: Systematic Review and Meta-Analysis: An overview with the help of R Software

Editor, International Journal of Statistics and Medical Informatics

1. Introduction
When a clinician wants to take a decision on a treatment, procedure or diagnosis with respect to a disease or condition, outcome from a single research may not be right or helpful. Systematic review provides the clinician with the strongest evidence about the available treatment or procedure related to a particular disease by including the evidences from the research studies which are similar in nature with respect to the scope, objective and the inclusion criteria of the study. Systematic reviews are different from the normal review or literature review as the later does not include all the relevant studies with respect to the particular problem and hence the conclusion drawn from it are not valid and generalizable. Meta-Analysis is a statistical tool helps us to combine the results from the studies under consideration and arrive at an aggregate value for the parameters under study such as odds ratio, survival rate etc. This chapter provides an overview of systematic review and meta-analysis

2. Systematic Review process
   i.   **Define research problem or question**
        Systematic review starts with the defining the research question based on Participants, Interventions, Comparison, Outcomes, Study design (PICOS)
   ii.   **Define objectives for the study**
        Develop objectives for the study which helps to focus on the research question or problem under study.
   iii.   **Define inclusion and exclusion criteria** [7]
        It allows us to select the studies for research question under study. Criteria includes the following parameters
          a. Study population
          b. Type of the studies (Randomized Control Studies, observational studies etc)
          c. Randomization methods

- d. Outcome measures
- e. Time period
- f. Sample size
- g. Patient characteristics

iv. **Define Search process**

The research papers can be searched through various

- a. Free databases such as PubMed, Cochrane Library, Google Scholar and also through Paid databases such as EMBASE, Psychinfo, NIAHL based on the type of the study question.
- b. Search for unpublished papers from the university and clinical repositories, conference proceedings
- c. During this phase of the systematic review there are possible bias can occur
    - i. Publication bias

      This is the most important bias in the process of systematic review which affects the quality of the review as a whole. Generally the studies with the positive results or outcome tend to be published more and studies with the negative results published rarely.
    - ii. Language Bias

      Majority of the journals or databases contains studies which are written in the English language and the papers written in the other languages tend to left out during the search process

v. **Select studies and evaluate the quality of selected studies**

Studies to be selected from the pool of studies obtained through the search process matching the including criteria and not fulfilling exclusion criteria. Further the studies to be evaluated for possible bias in study design, analytical tools, reporting structure, relevancy of the outcome measures etc.

vi. **Extract data**

Once the studies are selected and evaluated for possible bias, the next to step is to extract data from the selected for further processing

vii. **Synthesize the evidence**

Evidence from various can be synthesized or combined with or without the help of meta-analysis.

viii. **Meta-Analysis**

Meta-analysis helps to arrive at pooled estimates of outcomes measures such as odd ratio, survival rate or effect size.

The effect size is the standardized mean difference between the two groups [5]. Effect size is calculated from the difference between the mean of the treatment group and control group divided by the pooled standard deviation of the two groups. The effect size can be interpreted using the method suggested by Cohen [6] wherein if effect size is less than 0.2 it is interpreted as low, if it is between 0.2 and 0.5 it is interpreted as average and if it is above 0.8 it is interpreted as high.

Forest Plot

Forest plot is used to plot the effect size of outcomes measure with respect to each study. It also contains the overall effect size combined from for all the studies under review represented by black diamond shaped component in the bottom of the plot. Forest plot is vertically split into two portions one is for the control group and another is for the treatment group. If the effect size lines are there in the treatment group then it can be inferred that the treatment group is better than the control. If the black diamond is placed after 0.8 in the horizontal scale then the effect size is also high.

Funnel plot

Funnel plot helps us to detect any publication bias or heterogeneity in terms of the selected study by comparing the treatment effect against the precision of the selected studies. If a symmetric inverted funnel is obtained based on the data, then the systematic review does not have publication bias otherwise there is a possibility of publication bias or difference between the studies

ix. **Draw inferences, conclusion and report**
The last but the important step in the systematic review process is drawing inferences from the information summarized from the various studies and preparing the report.

3. Systematic Review Standards

The widely used and popular standards for systematic review are the Cochrane review standards [3]. Preferred Reporting Items for Systematic Reviews and Meta-Analysis (PRISMA) statement [4] helps us to provide guidelines on minimum set of items for reporting in systematic reviews and meta-analysis.

4. Illustrative Example

The following section provides an example for carrying out Systematic review and Meta-analysis. The main important point to be considered by the readers that the following example is just for illustrative purpose as it involves only few studies and the actual systematic review is more rigorous, voluminous and takes 8 months to 1 year to complete.

1. **Research problem**
   Is stent placement is effective than angioplasty in the treatment of coronary artery disease
2. **Objective of the study**
   To assess effect of the stent placement in comparison with the angioplasty in treating the coronary artery disease
3. **Inclusion criteria for studies**
   Studies which are comparing the effects of stent with the angioplasty in treating the coronary artery disease

Table-1 : Sample Inclusion criteria

Parameters	Inclusion Criteria
Study population	Ischemic heart disease and new lesions of the native coronary circulation
Treatment group	Stent
Control group	Angioplasty
Study design	RCT
Outcome measures	1. Procedural success 2. Reduction in stenosis 3. Survival rate 4. Myocardial infraction rate 5. CABG rate

Table-2: Sample Exclusion criteria

Parameters	Exclusion Criteria
Study population	1. Myocardial infraction within previous 7 days 2. Serious disease in left main coronary artery

4. **Search Process**

The following studies are retrieved from the google scholar and PubMed database based on the search term "Comparison of coronary-stent placement and balloon angioplasty in the treatment of coronary artery disease"

1. Fischman, D. L., Leon, M. B., Baim, D. S., Schatz, R. A., Savage, M. P., Penn, I., ... & Cleman, M. (1994). A randomized comparison of coronary-stent placement and balloon angioplasty in the treatment of coronary artery disease. *New England Journal of Medicine, 331*(8), 496-501.

2. Serruys, P. W., De Jaegere, P., Kiemeneij, F., Macaya, C., Rutsch, W., Heyndrickx, G., ... & Belardi, J. (1994). A comparison of balloon-expandable-stent implantation with balloon angioplasty in patients with coronary artery disease. New England Journal of Medicine, 331(8), 489-495.
3. Serruys, P. W., van Hout, B., Bonnier, H., Legrand, V., Garcia, E., Macaya, C., ... & Kiemeneij, F. (1998). Randomised comparison of implantation of heparin-coated stents with balloon angioplasty in selected patients with coronary artery disease (Benestent II). The Lancet, 352(9129), 673-681.
4. Betriu, A., Masotti, M., Serra, A., Alonso, J., Fernández-Avilés, F., Gimeno, F., ... & Calabuig, J. (1999). Randomized comparison of coronary stent implantation and balloon angioplasty in the treatment of de novo coronary artery lesions (START): a four-year follow-up. Journal of the American College of Cardiology, 34(5), 1498-1506.
5. Savage, M. P., Douglas Jr, J. S., Fischman, D. L., Pepine, C. J., King, S. B., Werner, J. A., ... & Leon, M. B. (1997). Stent placement compared with balloon angioplasty for obstructed coronary bypass grafts. New England Journal of Medicine, 337(11), 740-747.
6. Suryapranata, H., van't Hof, A. W., Hoorntje, J. C., de Boer, M. J., & Zijlstra, F. (1998). Randomized comparison of coronary stenting with balloon angioplasty in selected patients with acute myocardial infarction. Circulation, 97(25), 2502-2505.
7. Kastrati, A., Schömig, A., Dirschinger, J., Mehilli, J., Dotzer, F., von Welser, N., & Neumann, F. J. (2000). A randomized trial comparing stenting with balloon angioplasty in small vessels in patients with symptomatic coronary artery disease. Circulation, 102(21), 2593-2598.
8. Rubartelli, Paolo, Luigi Niccoli, Edoardo Verna, Corinna Giachero, Marco Zimarino, Alessandro Fontanelli,

Corrado Vassanelli et al. "Stent implantation versus balloon angioplasty in chronic coronary occlusions: results from the GISSOC trial." *Journal of the American College of Cardiology* 32, no. 1 (1998): 90-96.

9. Savage, M. P., Fischman, D. L., Rake, R., Leon, M. B., Schatz, R. A., Penn, I., ... & Baim, D. (1998). Efficacy of coronary stenting versus balloon angioplasty in small coronary arteries. *Journal of the American College of Cardiology, 31*(2), 307-311.

10. Versaci, F., Gaspardone, A., Tomai, F., Crea, F., Chiariello, L., & Gioffrè, P. A. (1997). A comparison of coronary-artery stenting with angioplasty for isolated stenosis of the proximal left anterior descending coronary artery. *New England Journal of Medicine, 336*(12), 817-822.

It is important to note that the above 10 studies are retrieved only from two databases (Google scholar and PubMed) with a basic search operation. In real time search more studies can be retrieved from the above mentioned databases as well as other databases such as EMBASE and NIAHL etc.

5. **Selection of Studies**

    The above studies to be evaluated for matching the inclusion criteria and also those studies which are matching inclusion criteria should not match the exclusion criteria. The studies 1 and 4 can be included from the above set of studies for further analysis (only for illustrative purpose. The two selected studies evaluated for possible bias such study design and sample size. Both the studies used the RCT and it was explicitly mentioned. Though the sample size is different for the studies, it is acceptable (205 vs 229). The outcomes measures such as

    Procedural success, diameter of the lumen, restenosis rate, survival rate, myocardial infraction rate, CABG rate etc are also defined in both the studies

It is important to note that the two studies are selected and evaluated for possible bias with few parameters only for the illustrative purpose. In real time analysis more studies can be included and evaluated before proceeding to the next step.

6. **Extraction of data**

   The following data needs to be extracted from the two studies for synthesizing the information from the two studies (but not limited to) and the data extracted is only for illustrative purpose

   i. **Study citation**

      a. @article{fischman1994randomized,
         title={A randomized comparison of coronary-stent placement and balloon angioplasty in the treatment of coronary artery disease},
         author={Fischman, David L and Leon, Martin B and Baim, Donald S and Schatz, Richard A and Savage, Michael P and Penn, Ian and Detre, Katherine and Veltri, Lisa and Ricci, Donald and Nobuyoshi, Masakiyo and others},
         journal={New England Journal of Medicine},
         volume={331},
         number={8},
         pages={496--501},
         year={1994},
         publisher={Mass Medical Soc}}

      b. @article{betriu1999randomized,
         title={Randomized comparison of coronary stent implantation and balloon angioplasty in the treatment of de novo coronary artery lesions (START): a four-year follow-up},

```
author={Betriu, Amadeo and Masotti, Monica
and Serra, Antoni and Alonso, Joaquin and
Fern{\'a}ndez-Avil{\'e}s, Francisco and Gimeno,
Federico and Colman, Thierry and Zueco, Javier
and Delcan, Juan L and Garc{\i}a, Eulogio and
others},
journal={Journal of the American College of
Cardiology},
volume={34},
number={5},
pages={1498--1506},
year={1999},
publisher={Elsevier}
}
```

ii. **Sample size**
Study 1 – Stent group – 205, Balloon Angioplasty group - 202
Study 2 – Stent group -229, Balloon Angioplasty group - 223

iii. **Duration of the study**
Study1 - Six months
Study2- Four years (Duration of the study varies significantly)

iv. **Follow up period**
Study1 – Six months (restenosis)
Study2 – Six months (restenosis),Four years for death, myocardial infarction (MI) and target vessel revascularization (Follow up period varies significantly)

v. **Analytical tool used**
Study-1
Continuous data – two tailed t test was used to test the difference between the sample means
Categorical data - Chi-Square test was used
Composite clinical end point – Kaplan Meir survival curve with Wilcoxon test to test the difference between the two means

Study-2

Continuous data – two tailed t test was used to test the difference between the sample means

Categorical data - Chi-Square test was used. For discrete variables Fisher's Exact test is used

Comparison of treatment means – Relative Risk with confidence interval used

Composite clinical end point – Kaplan Meir survival curve with log rank statistics to test the difference between the two means

vi. **Outcome measures**

Table-3: Sample Outcome Measures

	Study 1 Stent group	Angioplasty group	Study 2 Stent group	Angioplasty group
Procedural success	96.1%	89.6%	95%	84%
Increase in the Diameter of the luman	1.72±0.46mm	1.23±0.48mm	2.02±0.6mm	1.43±0.6mm
Restenosis rate	31.6%	42.1%	22%	37%
Coronary related disease rate	19.5%	23.8%	2.2%	2.8%
Revascularization rate	10.2%	15.4%	12%	25%

vii. **Results and conclusion**

Stent was effective in both the studies than the Balloon Angioplasty

viii. **Meta-Analysis**
Effect size of the outcome measures is calculated and forest and funnel plot are plotted as below
This paper uses R software [8] to carry out the Meta-analysis. R is open source statistical software and it includes number of packages developed by the R community for specific purposes. R – Studio [9] is a widely used environment for executing R codes. This paper uses the following R packages for carrying out the Meta-Analysis which needs to be installed through R-Studio.

R package – Metafor[10]
It includes functions and plots to carry out Meta-analysis

The R code for calculating the effect size, forest plot and funnel plot is given below:
##install metafor package
Install.packages(metafor)
install xlsx package to import excel extracted data set to r environment, The excel data set contains the following variable Study , Sample size, Mean and standard deviation of increase in size of luman for 8 sample studies

1. sno
2. study
3. s_samplesize_s
4. s_luman_mean
5. s_luman_std
6. a_samplesize_s
7. a_luman_mean
8. a_luman_stda

install.packages(xlsx)
# Load package metafor and xlsx
library(metafor)
library(xlsx)

Read data from metadata.xlsx from c directory with first row contains the variable name

```
mydata <- read.xlsx("C:/metadata.xlsx", 1)
##Calculate effect size using mean difference
effect  <-  rma(m1  =  s_luman_mean,  m2  =  a_luman_mean,
                sd1 = s_luman_std, sd2 = a_luman_stda,
                n1 = s_samplesize_s, n2 = a_samplesize_s,
                method = "FE", measure = "MD",
                data = mydata)
##Plot forest plot
forest(effect)
##Plot funnel plot
funnel(result.md)
```

Output

The forest plot is shown in the below chart-1

Chart-1: Forest Plot

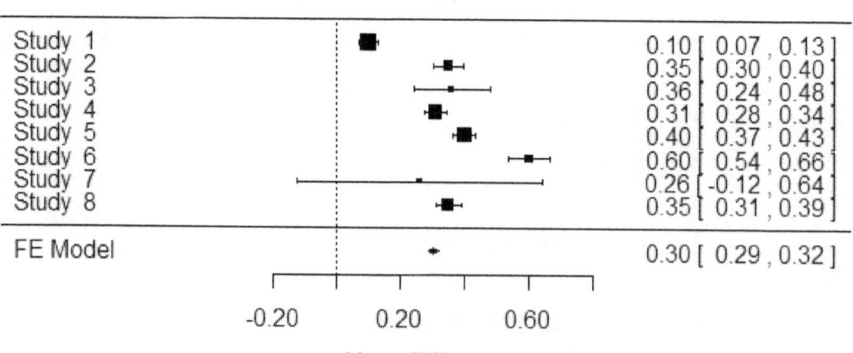

The forest plot gives the effect size on the increase in luman size with respect to the stent group in comparison with angioplasty group. The right side of forest plot belongs to the stent group and left hand side belongs to the angioplasty group. It can be inferred that all lines are in the right hand side indicating the stent group is effective than the angioplasty group. The black diamond falls between 0.2 and 0.6, indicating the effect size is average.
The following chart-2 provides Funnel plot

Chart-2: Funnel Plot

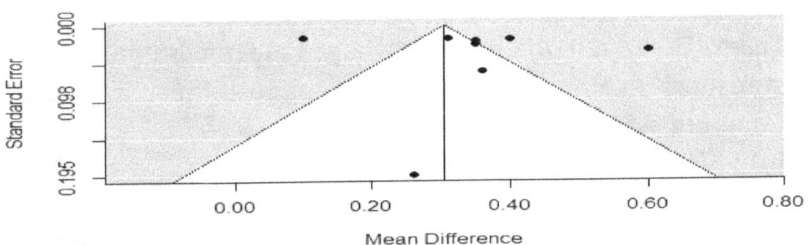

The above chart shows there is a bias in the data which may be due to publication bias as the mean difference values does not fall into the inverted funnel area

Conclusion
This Chapter provided an overview of systematic review and meta-analysis. An illustrative example is used to explain the systematic review and meta-analysis process and m eta-analysis was carried out using the R statistical software.

References
1. Khan, K. S., Kunz, R., Kleijnen, J., & Antes, G. (2003). Five steps to conducting a systematic review. *Journal of the Royal Society of Medicine, 96*(3), 118-121.
2. Centre for reviews, & dissemination (CRD). (2009). *Systematic reviews: CRD's guidance for undertaking reviews in health care.* Centre for Reviews and Dissemination.

3. Higgins JPT, Green S (editors). COCHRANE HANDBOOK FOR SYSTEMATIC REVIEWS OF INTERVENTIONS Version 5.1.0 [updated March 2011]. The Cochrane Collaboration, 2011. Available from http://handbook.cochrane.org.
4. http://www.prisma-statement.org/
5. Coe, R. (2002). It's the effect size, stupid: What effect size is and why it is important.
6. Cohen, J. (1977). Statistical power analysis for the behavioural sciences (Revised edition). *New York, 7*.
7. Meline, T. (2006). Selecting studies for systematic review: Inclusion and exclusion criteria. *Contemporary issues in communication science and disorders, 33*(21-27).
8. Team, R. C. (2014). R: A language and environment for statistical computing. R Foundation for Statistical Computing, Vienna, Austria. 2013.
9. https://www.rstudio.com/
10. ByteCompile, T. R. U. E., & LazyData, T. R. U. E. (2016). Package 'metafor'.

Chapter2: Structural Equation Modelling in the biomedical domain: Concepts and methods revisited with the help of statistical package

Editor, International Journal of Statistics and Medical Informatics

1. Introduction

Structural Equation Modelling (SEM) is widely used in the social sciences [1, 2] analysing complex relationships among multiple variables. It is defined by two models measurement model and construct model. Measurement model defines the relationship between observed variables and constructs (or latent variables or factors or unobserved variables) which are derived from observed variables. Construct model defines the relationship between the construct or latent variables. SEM is able to model the error terms in the observed variables and error while defining the relationship in the model and it is a unique property of SEM. The objective of SEM is to verify whether a model specified prior is a best fit to the given data or not. This chapter provides an overview of Structural Equation Modelling, its application in biomedical domain and illustrated with the help of R Statistical Software.

2. Architecture of Structural Equation Model

The architecture of the SEM [3] is given in the figure-1 below and it contains two models namely measurement model and construct model. The measurement defines the relationship between Measurement variables M1, M2 with Latent variable L1 similarly measurement variables M3 and M4 with L2 along with associated measurement errors E1 &E2 and E3 & E4 respectively. It also contains the construct model which defines the relationship between the Latent variables L1 and L2 along with the associated error variable LE1

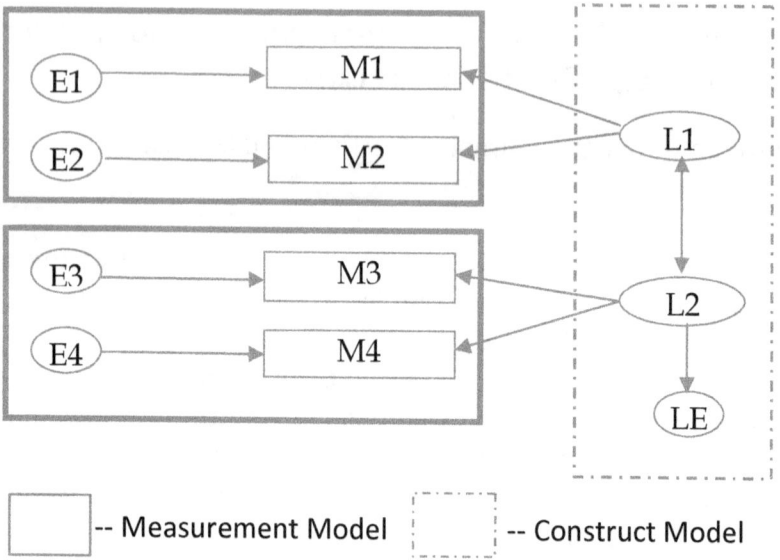

☐ -- Measurement Model   ⁝ ⁝ -- Construct Model

Figure -1: Architecture of SEM
M1 – Measurement Variable1
E1 – Error associated with Measurement Variable M1
L1 – Latent variable 1 derived from the linear combination of Measurement Variable M1 and M2
LE1 – Error Associated with Latent Variable L1

3. **Mediation and Moderation effect**
   i. Mediation effect [4] acts like a mediator between independent and dependent variable and influences the relationship between the independent and dependent variable. Mediation effect is also termed as indirect effect is given in the figure-2 below:

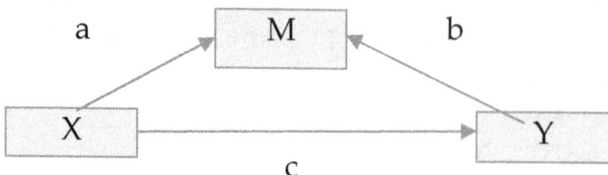

Figure-2: Mediator effect

Here X – independent variable
Y – Dependent Variable
M – Mediator variable
c – Direct effect
a, b – indirect effect

ii. Moderator effect [4] modifies the casual relationship between independent and dependent variable. It modifies the strength and direction of the relationship between dependent variable which is depicted in the figure-3 below:

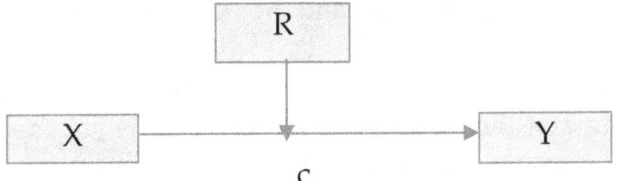

Figure-3: Moderator effect

Here X – independent variable
Y – Dependent Variable
R – Moderator variable
c – Effect modified by Moderator variable

4. **Comparison between SEM and Traditional Model**

The comparison between SEM and Traditional Statistical Models is given in the below Table-1.

Table-1 Comparison between SEM and Traditional Statistical Models

Description	SEM	Traditional Statistical Models
variables	Measured and latent variables	Measured variables
Specification of Model	Model to be specified priory	Model to be derived
Input Data	Variance Covariance matrix as data input	Raw Data as data input

5. **Steps in building Structural Equation Modelling**
   The building of SEM involves certain defined steps [5] such as specification, identification, estimation of the model and computation of goodness of fit for the model.
   a. **Specification of the model**
      Model specification is the first step wherein the relationship between measurement variables and latent variables to be specified and also the relationship among the latent variables needs to be specified. This step requires a prior knowledge about the research problem and the research area.
   b. **Identification of the model**
      Model identification involves finding unique solutions to the parameters of the model. The solution can be just identified (one solution for each parameter), under identified (infinite number of solution for each parameter) and over identified (more than one solution with one optimum solution)
   c. **Estimation of the model**
      There are several estimation methods available to estimate the variance and covariance matrix such as Maximum Likelihood, Least Square, Asymptotically distribution Free estimation methods. Maximum Likelihood estimation is widely used method to estimate the variance-covariance matrix. The drawback of this method is it requires large sample size. Least Square method overcomes the drawback of large sample size and it works well with the smaller sample size also
   d. **Computation of goodness of fit**
      Goodness of fit of the developed model is tested using the chi-square statistics and if we obtain the non-significant value of Chi-Square statistics then the model is a good fit to the given data
      The Chi-Square tests the difference between variance covariance estimated by the model vs variance and covariance observed from the data.

6. **Application of SEM in Biomedical Domain [6, 7]**
   SEM is used to study the patient behavioural aspects [8, 9], relationship between life style & health condition [10, 11] and risk factors associated with disease [12, 13]. SEM is also used in the field of epidemiology [14]. The application in the biomedical field is still less compared to other fields such as social sciences.

7. **Advantages and Disadvantages of SEM**
   i. **Advantages**
      a. Simultaneously testing parameters at the individual at the model level
      b. Model assumptions are clearly specified before the estimation model
      c. Errors are measured at the measurement level and construct level
      d. Used to fit longitudinal models such as time series models.

   ii. **Disadvantages**
      a. It requires usually large sample size
      b. Derivation of Latent variable from the measurement variables is approximate

8. **Software available to SEM**
   SEM can be carried out using Statistical Analysis System (SAS) [15], Statistical Software for Social Sciences (SPSS) – AMOS [16], R Statistical Software [17]

9. **Illustrative example**
   SEM is illustrated using the R Statistical Software [17] which is open source Statistical software to analyse the risk factors associated with the congenital heart disease through a hypothetical dataset.

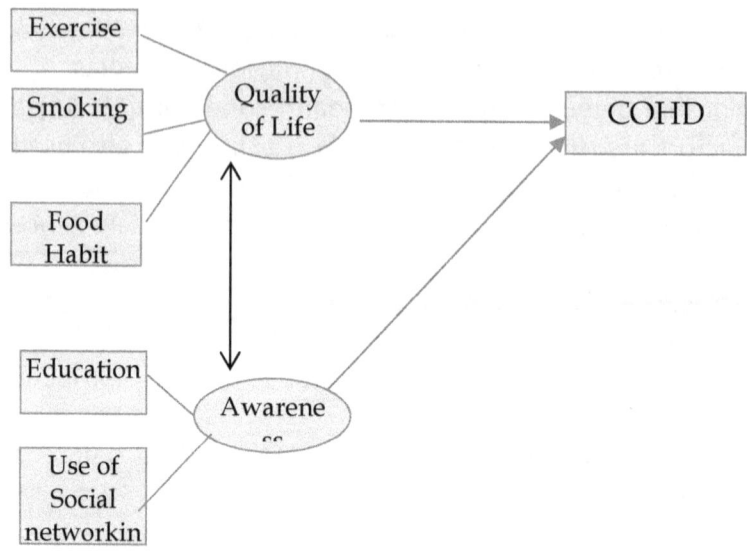

Rcode

Step-1

Set the working directory

```
>wd = "c://users//SEM"
>setwd(wd)
```

Step-2

Install lavaan package and import into r environment

```
>library(lavaan)
```

Step-3

Read the CSV data file and name the fields

```
>path1 = read.csv ("SEMsam.csv", header=FALSE)

>names(path1) = c("cohd", "exercise",
            "smoking","foodhab","edu","social","quality","aware")
```

Step-4

Build the model using model statement

```
>model <- '
  # measurement model
  quality =~ exercise + smoking + foodhab
  aware =~ edu + social
```

```
# regressions
cohd ~ quality + aware
quality ~ aware
# residual correlations
exercise ~~ foodhab
edu ~~ social
'
```

Step-5:
Fit the model with the sem statement
>fit = sem(model, data = path1, missing = 'listwise',se = 'bootstrap', bootstrap = 50)

Step-6:
Display the summary using summary statement
>summary(fit,fit.measures=TRUE, rsquare=TRUE, standardized=TRUE)

Output

lavaan (0.5-23.1097) converged normally after 84 iterations

Number of observations	300
Estimator	ML
Minimum Function Test Statistic	1.147
Degrees of freedom	5
P-value (Chi-square)	0.950

Model test baseline model:

Minimum Function Test Statistic	12.434
Degrees of freedom	15
P-value	0.646

User model versus baseline model:

Comparative Fit Index (CFI)	1.000
Tucker-Lewis Index (TLI)	-3.505

Loglikelihood and Information Criteria:

Loglikelihood user model (H0)	NA
Loglikelihood unrestricted model (H1)	NA
Number of free parameters	16
Akaike (AIC)	NA
Bayesian (BIC)	NA

Root Mean Square Error of Approximation:

RMSEA	0.000
90 Percent Confidence Interval	0.000 0.002
P-value RMSEA <= 0.05	0.990

Standardized Root Mean Square Residual:

SRMR	0.014

Parameter Estimates:

Information	Observed
Standard Errors	Bootstrap
Number of requested bootstrap draws	5
Number of successful bootstrap draws	4

Latent Variables:

	Estimate	Std.Err	z-value	P(>|z|)	Std.lv	Std.all
quality =~						
exercise	1.000				0.109	0.215
smoking	0.498	0.261	1.909	0.056	0.054	0.107
foodhab	0.762	0.404	1.889	0.059	0.083	0.164
aware =~						
edu	1.000				0.560	0.674
social	-0.201	0.338	-0.595	0.552	-0.112	-0.222

Regressions:

	Estimate	Std.Err	z-value	P(>|z|)	Std.lv	Std.all
cohd ~						
quality	2.667	186.501	0.014	0.989	0.291	0.574
aware	-0.271	0.044	-6.131	0.000	-0.152	-0.300
quality ~						
aware	0.078	0.052	1.491	0.136	0.399	0.399

Covariances:

	Estimate	Std.Err	z-value	P(>|z|)	Std.lv	Std.all
.exercise ~~						
.foodhab	0.018	0.010	1.780	0.075	0.018	0.072
.edu ~~						
.social	0.065	13.080	0.005	0.996	0.065	0.215

Variances:

	Estimate	Std.Err	z-value	P(>|z|)	Std.lv	Std.all
.exercise	0.244	0.016	14.944	0.000	0.244	0.954
.smoking	0.254	0.006	40.492	0.000	0.254	0.988
.foodhab	0.250	0.006	41.220	0.000	0.250	0.973
.edu	0.376	31.476	0.012	0.990	0.376	0.545
.social	0.244	5.397	0.045	0.964	0.244	0.951
.cohd	0.184	3.417	0.054	0.957	0.184	0.718
.quality	0.010	0.013	0.767	0.443	0.841	0.841
aware	0.313	31.490	0.010	0.992	1.000	1.000

R-Square:

	Estimate
exercise	0.046
smoking	0.012
foodhab	0.027
edu	0.455
social	0.049
cohd	0.282
quality	0.159

Discussion

The non-significant value of the chi-square statistics indicates that the model fits the data with R square value for the parameter education which is higher than the other parameters.

Conclusion

This Chapter provided an overview of Structural Equation Modelling in the biomedical domain with the help of R Statistical Package.

References

1. Ullman, J. B., & Bentler, P. M. (2003). Structural equation modelling. John Wiley & Sons, Inc..

2. Hox, J. J., & Bechger, T. M. (1998). An introduction to structural equation modelling.

3. Schumacker, R. E., & Lomax, R. G. (2004). *A beginner's guide to structural equation modeling.* psychology press

4. Wu, A. D., & Zumbo, B. D. (2008). Understanding and using mediators and moderators. *Social Indicators Research, 87*(3), 367.

5. Weston, R., & Gore Jr, P. A. (2006). A brief guide to structural equation modeling. *The counseling psychologist, 34*(5), 719-751.

6. Zhang, Z. (2017). Structural equation modelling in the context of clinical research. Annals of translational medicine, 5(5).

7. Beran, T. N., & Violato, C. (2010). Structural equation modelling in medical research: a primer. BMC research notes, 3(1), 267.

8. Holmes, C. S., Chen, R., Streisand, R., Marschall, D. E., Souter, S., Swift, E. E., & Peterson, C. C. (2005). Predictors of youth diabetes care behaviors and metabolic control: a structural equation modeling approach. *Journal of pediatric psychology, 31*(8), 770-784

9. Bol, Y., Duits, A. A., Lousberg, R., Hupperts, R. M., Lacroix, M. H., Verhey, F. R., & Vlaeyen, J. W. (2010). Fatigue and physical disability in patients with multiple sclerosis: a structural equation modeling approach. *Journal of behavioral medicine, 33*(5), 355-363.

10. Höfer, S., Benzer, W., Alber, H., Ruttmann, E., Kopp, M., Schussler, G., & Doering, S. (2005). Determinants of health-related quality of life in coronary artery disease patients: a prospective study generating a structural equation model. *Psychosomatics, 46*(3), 212-223.

11. Lee, J. W., Lee, K. E., Park, D. J., Kim, S. H., Nah, S. S., Lee, J. H., ... & Lee, H. S. (2017). Determinants of quality of life in patients with fibromyalgia: A structural equation modeling approach. *PloS one, 12*(2), e0171186.

12. Roman-Urrestarazu, A., Ali, F. M. H., Reka, H., Renwick, M. J., Roman, G. D., & Mossialos, E. (2016). Structural equation model for estimating risk factors in type 2 diabetes mellitus in a Middle Eastern setting: evidence from the STEPS Qatar. *BMJ Open Diabetes Research and Care, 4*(1), e000231.

13. Bardenheier, B. H., Bullard, K. M., Caspersen, C. J., Cheng, Y. J., Gregg, E. W., & Geiss, L. S. (2013). A novel use of structural equation models to examine factors associated with prediabetes among adults aged 50 years and older: National Health and Nutrition Examination Survey 2001–2006. *Diabetes care, 36*(9), 2655-2662.

14. Amorim, L. D. A. F., Fiaccone, R. L., Santos, C. A. S., Santos, T. N. D., de Moraes, L. T. L., Oliveira, N. F., ... & Barreto, M. L. (2010). Structural equation modeling in epidemiology. *Cadernos de Saúde Pública, 26*(12), 2251-2262.

15. O'Rourke, N., Psych, R., & Hatcher, L. (2013). *A step-by-step approach to using SAS for factor analysis and structural equation modeling*. Sas Institute.

16. Byrne, B. M. (2016). *Structural equation modelling with AMOS: Basic concepts, applications, and programming.* Routledge.

17. Fox, J. (2006). Teacher's corner: structural equation modelling with the sem package in R. *Structural equation modelling, 13*(3), 465-486.

Chapter3: An overview of clinical trial data management, its standards and recent trends

Editor, International Journal of Statistics and Medical Informatics

1. Introduction

Clinical trials help pharmaceutical/biomedical organisations to bring the drug/treatment/procedure from the development stage to the end user stage. Normally clinical trials consists of four stages Phase I – IV. During the Phase-III which involves human beings as the subject of trial, requires significant amount of data to be captured, cleaned, transformed, compiled, audited, analysed and reported. Traditional data management techniques may not be sufficient to manage the current clinical trials as they are conducted at different location results in high cost of collecting, storing and processing of data. Hence there is need for advanced technologies such as online/web based data management techniques to increase the efficiency in collecting, storing and processing of data and also to reduce the cost related to the clinical trial data. This chapter starts with a brief overview of clinical trials, regulatory requirement, guidelines, and its different phases. It further discusses the traditional tools, techniques and standards to handle clinical trials data, software available for clinical trial data management and recent trends.

2. Clinical Trials

Clinical trials are experiments conducted to study the efficacy and safety aspects of a drug/treatment/procedure which may or may not involve human being as the subject for the study [1]. The human beings involved in the study may be normal/healthy human beings or affected by a disease or condition. Clinical trial tries to provide solution to scientific questions and prevent or treat a disease or condition [2]. Clinical trials are conducted as a single centre or multicentre trial based on the requirement.

3. Food and Drug Administration (FDA)

Once the study is over, findings of the study are submitted to regulatory authorities for approval. In United States of America (USA), the Food and Drug Administration's [FDA] Centre for Drug Evaluation and Research (CDER) gives the final approval before it is marketed in USA while ensuring the new drug is safe and effective [3]. The application procedure for a new drug can be referred at FDA webpage [4]

4. International Council for Harmonization (ICH)

Clinical trials involving medications/drugs are guided by International Council for Harmonisation (ICH) guideline for good clinical practice [5]. It aims to achieve harmonization at the global level to ensure the safe, effective and high quality medications [6]. Current ICH guidelines includes four categories namely quality, efficacy, safety and multidisciplinary guidelines

5. Trial Protocols

Clinical trials includes protocol[7] or plan which includes the trial background, objectives, design, patient recruitment, ethical consideration, adverse event reporting, study sample size and randomization schedule and statistical analysis. A sample trial protocol related to the University of Nottingham's Controlled Assessment of Salicylates and Azathioprine (CASA trial) can be referred at the trial's website [8]

6. Different phases of clinical trial

Clinical trial related to development of new drug for a specific disease or condition normally consists of four phases namely phase I-IV [9] which is described in the Table-1 below:

Table-1: Clinical Trial Phases

Phases	Objective	Approximate number of study participants required	Type of study participants
Phase-I	To study the safety of the drug and determine the dosage of the proposed new drug	Less than 20	Most likely severely ill patients
Phase-II	To study the primary outcome (efficacy) in relation to the new drug under consideration. It also continue to study the safety aspect also	Less than or equal to 100	Patients with the disease or condition
Phase III	To study effect of new drug in comparison to the standard drug. It involves one or more group of patients wherein the new and standard drug is administered with the use of randomization schedule. It might be single centre or multi-centre study. It is usually includes at least two phase III trials which are required to confirm the effectiveness of the new drug	Less than or equal to 1000	Patients with the disease or condition.

| Phase IV | To study side effect of the new drug and it is a post marketing surveillance study after regulatory approval is obtained | Less than or equal to 10000 | General Population |

During the pre-clinical trial phase pharmacodynamics and pharmacokinetics are parameters are determined for the drug and it mostly involve animals [9, 10].

7. Clinical Trial Data Management (CTDM)

Clinical Trial Data Management (CDTM) takes centre stage throughout the clinical trial process especially in the phase III of the clinical trial. Basic or Standard CTDM involves the following components [11]

a. Case Report Form (CRF) and its annotation

Case report from is a basic instrument used to collect the data for the clinical trial. The case report form's structured format helps the researchers to ensure the quality of the data collected. Case report form is prepared based on the clinical trial protocol and it adheres to the data validity requirements. The CRFs can be a prepared as simple manual form or web based online form which is useful in the case of multi central trials to make the data collection uniform across the centres. Data in the CRF are entered by the trained users and usually data entry errors are controlled by the automated validation at the form level itself such as preventing format errors such as text in the date field (Date of Birth will allow only the date of birth in the dd/mm/yyyy format) or the maximum/minimum value for a particular field or closed ended fields.

Annotated CRF provides details about where the data is stored or path of the data with respect to each section of the CRF so that every researcher who is involved in the trial has knowledge about the storage of data.

b. Data validation
Once the data is stored in the database, data is to be validated against the set protocol of the clinical trial. The CRFs which confirms to the validation requirement only be processed for the next level.

c. Data Auditing
Data to be audited for any deviation found in the data and if it is found, it should be recorded with reason for deviation.

d. Clinical Coding
Standard Clinical Terminologies to be used when representing the diseases, drugs and other clinical parameters.

e. Database freezing
Once data is validated and audited, the database is to be locked before the start of the statistical analysis to ensure the validity results.

8. CDISC – Clinical Data Interchange Standards Consortium
Clinical Data Interchange Standards Consortium (CDISC) is a non-governmental organization which aims to develop and support global, platform-independent data standards that enable information system interoperability to improve medical research and related areas of healthcare [12]. The standards has [13,14] foundational standards, and data exchange standards which covers the different stages of clinical trials starting from the planning stage to the data analysis stage including the data exchange part. The following Table-2 provides the details about CDISC

Table-2: Clinical Data Interchange Standards Consortium (CDISC)

Standards	Components	Elements	Description
Foundational Standards	Planning	Protocol	Provides standard format for study protocol
		Study Design	Provides formats of interchangeable and machine readable study designs

	Data collection	Clinical Data Acquisition Standards Harmonization (CDASH)	Defines set of data collection elements formats
		Laboratory Data Model (LAB)	Defines formats for transferring data between laboratory and study site
	Data tabulation	Study Data Tabulation Model (SDTM) Standard Exchange Of Non-Clinical Data (SEND)	Provides formats for tabulation data it contains three main classes namely events, intervention and findings in a trial
	Statistical Analysis	Analysis Data Model (ADaM)	Provides data structure for analysis. It contains three classes namely Subject Level Data Analysis, Basic Data Structure and Adverse Event Analysis Dataset
Data Exchange Standards	Data Transfer	Study/ Trial Design Model - eXtensible Markup Language (SDM-XML)	Used to transfer data between organizations using XML
		Operational Data Model	Provides standards for data transfer
		Define eXtensible Markup Language (XML)	Describes the metadata during the transfer

9. Software used in Clinical Trial Data Management – Electronic Data Capture (EDC)/Clinical Data Management Solutions(CDMS)

The following table provides details of software available to manage the data in a clinical trial

Software	Description	Link
SAS	Commercial Package	www.sas.com
Velos	Commercial Package	http://velos.com/velos-eresearch
Medidata Rave	Commercial Package	https://www.mdsol.com/en/products/rave
Openclinica	Open source software	https://www.openclinica.com/
ONCORE	University of Wisconsin Institute for Clinical and Translational Research software	https://ictr.wisc.edu/oncore/
WebDCU™ system.	Medical University of South Carolina web based software	https://dcu.musc.edu/Solution/WebDCUoverview.aspx
REdcap	Available free for institutions that join the REDCap Consortium.	https://projectredcap.org/software/
CTMS	Mayo Clinic 's Clinical Trial Management System (restricted access)	http://www.mayo.edu/research/labs/clinical-trials-management-system/about
Penn CTMS	University of Pennsylvania Clinical Trial Management System (restricted access)	http://www.med.upenn.edu/ocr/about-ctms.html

10. Latest Trend in Clinical Trial Data management

The clinical trial data management has evolved over time from using manual collect and analyse data(paper based) to capturing the data electronically and analysing the data using advanced statistical software. Currently the emergence of technology tools such as wearable device, eSource technology, emergence of cloud computing, text mining and social media have greater impact on the clinical trial data management in terms of reduced time, tasks and cost [15].

a. eSource Technology

eSource technology helps to electronically capture the patient data. Patient measurements are directly fed into eCRF without the need of manual entry into CRF. Real time data collection is possible with the help of eSource technology and it helps in avoiding duplication of data, reducing the data entry time and data entry errors [16]

b. Electronic Patient Reported Outcome (ePRO)

Electronic Patient reported outcomes helps to achieve more accuracy and compliance in the data collection and reducing the duplication of data [17]. The ePRO are collected through the devices provided by the clinical trial organizations with the required software or bring your own devices approach for study participants to report the outcomes.

c. Wearable devices

Wearable devices such as wristbands, clothing tags monitor and collects the data related patients vital signs and physical activities respectively in a real time environment [18, 19]. It helps in reducing time, cost and repeated visit of patient to the clinical trial site

d. Cloud Computing

Cloud computing technology provides reduced Information Technology infrastructure requirement through the shared pool of computing resources such as servers and databases. Some of the benefit of the cloud computing are it is available as service, available everywhere and scalability. Clinical trial organizations are yet to adopt the technology

fully due to the factors such as security and lack of control [20]
   e. **Use of social networks**
      Social media groups are useful in providing awareness about the disease or its treatment. It also helps in recruiting study participants for a clinical trial [21]

11. Conclusion
    This chapter provided an overview of clinical trial, data management in clinical trial, related standards, software used in clinical trial data management and the recent trends in clinical trial data management

References
1. https://www.nhlbi.nih.gov/studies/clinicaltrials
2. https://medlineplus.gov/clinicaltrials.html
3. https://www.fda.gov/drugs/developmentapprovalprocess/howdrugsaredevelopedandapproved/
4. https://www.fda.gov/drugs/developmentapprovalprocess/howdrugsaredevelopedandapproved/approvalapplications/newdrugapplicationnda/default.htm
5. http://www.ich.org/about/mission.html
6. https://www.ich.org/fileadmin/Public_Web_Site/ICH_Products/Guidelines/Efficacy/E6/E6_R1_Guideline.pdf
7. Bellomo, R., Weinberg, L., & Armellini, A. (2014). CLINICAL TRIAL PROTOCOL.
8. Logan, R. F. A. CLINICAL TRIAL PROTOCOL. *Assessment*, 9(10), 10.
9. https://onlinecourses.science.psu.edu/stat509/node/22
10. Mahan, V. L. (2014). Clinical trial phases. *International Journal of Clinical Medicine*, 5(21), 1374.
11. Krishnankutty, B., Bellary, S., Kumar, N. B., & Moodahadu, L. S. (2012). Data management in clinical research: an overview. *Indian journal of pharmacology*, 44(2), 168.
12. https://www.cdisc.org/about/what-we-do
13. Sandra Minjoe, PharmaSUG 2013 - Paper IB06 Introduction to the CDISC Standards

14. de Montjoie, A. J. (2009). *Introducing the CDISC standards: new efficiencies for medical research*. CDISC.
15. Henderson, L. (2017). The Clinical Trial of Tomorrow. *Applied Clinical Trials, 25*(2/3), 6.
16. Nordo, A. H., Eisenstein, E. L., Hawley, J., Vadakkeveedu, S., Pressley, M., Pennock, J., & Sanderson, I. (2017). A comparative effectiveness study of eSource used for data capture for a clinical research registry. *International Journal of Medical Informatics, 103*, 89-94.
17. Coons, S. J., Eremenco, S., Lundy, J. J., O'Donohoe, P., O'Gorman, H., & Malizia, W. (2015). Capturing patient-reported outcome (PRO) data electronically: the past, present, and promise of ePRO measurement in clinical trials. The Patient-Patient-Centered Outcomes Research, 8(4), 301-309.
18. Owens, S. (2017). Wearable Devices in Clinical Trials: The Opportunities and Challenges. *Neurology Today, 17*(14), 24-27.
19. Blackman, N. M. D. (2016). The Growing Availability of Wearable Devices: A Perspective on Current Applications in Clinical Trials.
20. Ohmann, C., Canham, S., Danielyan, E., Robertshaw, S., Legré, Y., Clivio, L., & Demotes, J. (2015). 'Cloud computing'and clinical trials: report from an ECRIN workshop. *Trials, 16*(1), 318.
21. Shere, M., Zhao, X. Y., & Koren, G. (2014). The role of social media in recruiting for clinical trials in pregnancy. *PloS one, 9*(3), e92744.

Chapter4: Natural Language Processing concepts and methods revisited

Editor, International Journal of Statistics and Medical Informatics

1. Introduction

Natural Language Processing [1,2] (NLP) evolved from the field computational linguistics which includes methods to study the language with the help of computers. It started with the process of translating languages [3] into another language with the use of machine translations algorithms. At next level, computers started understanding the language by parsing the sentences and deriving meaning out of the sentences. Moving further in this direction, rule based algorithms used in the next stage following statistical methods are used to process the language. Ambiguity in the natural languages is still a hurdle for the NLP systems even though lot work has been done to reduce the ambiguities. Statistical methods can help us to resolve ambiguities and learning from the set of data or corpus.

Usage of NLP systems in biomedical domain [4] is increasing as there is a need to understand the hidden knowledge in the vast text document present in the biomedical literature

2. Applications of NLP in Biomedical domain

NLP is used to extract information from the Electronic Medical Records [5], encoding of clinical documents [6], clinical decision support [7,8], and disease status identification [9,10] in combination with text mining

3. General Applications of NLP

NLP based applications are used in the fields of Machine Translation[3], dialog systems, Information retrieval, Information extraction, Named Entity Recognition, Question Answering and Sentiment Analysis[11].

4. Basic language terms and definitions used in Natural Language Processing

The Table-1 below provides commonly used basic terms and definitions in NLP systems which give the users fair idea about the system.

Table 1 – Basic Terms and Definitions in NLP

Terms	Definitions
Semantics	Meaning of words
Morpheme	Sub part of the words which has meaning
Bag of words	Frequency of words
String of words	Linear sequence of words
Tree of words	Represented by recursive structure of language
Word Boundary	Space between words
Word formation	Inflection, Derivation and Compounding
Sentences boundary	Formed by full stop and semicolon
Syntax	Rules to form sentences from words(Grammar).
Parsing/Part of Speech tagging/Chunking	Dividing the sentences into parts using syntactic structure/Grammar
Text categorization	Assigning documents to predetermined list of topics
Lexicon	Dictionary or list of words
Tokenization	Divided the text into smaller units of words, numbers or punctuation
Discourse	Analysing the two or more connected sentences in a given text or document
Pragmatic	Analysing the text in context of world knowledge

5. **Approaches to NLP [12]**
    i. Linguistic approach

Linguistic approach uses rule based approach wherein the set of rules are applied on given input and the rule which matches the condition is executed.

   ii. Statistical approach

Statistical approach uses statistical models such as Hidden Markov Models wherein the models is defined by a set of states and its associated transition probabilities when the transition happens from state to another state. The states are hidden in the Models but output of each transition is observable with certain probabilities

6. **Text Classification[13]**

6.1 Supervised Classification

During the training phase a set of features is extracted from the input and then label is assigned to each feature which acts as a classifier. Once the new input text is fed into the classifier and a set of features are extracted from the given new input. Now classifier assigns label to new input using the training set and the same is added into training set for future classifications.

Examples of supervised classification can be seen in assigning topics to given input or labelling a given text input as positive or negative sentiments or classifying an email as spam or not spam

6.1.1. Naïve Bayes classifier

Naïve Bayes classifier [13] uses prior probabilities to assign label to a given input through the features and associated feature weight for the each label in the training set.

For example consider a case when an article which needs to classified into a particular topic using the Naïve Bayes classifier. Our training classifier contains documents related to diseases such as cancer, diabetes mellitus, and arterial disease, feature set and corresponding labels. If the input article is on cancer then the classifier starts extracting features from the given article which contains more features related to cancer and more weight will be given to the features related to the cancer during the classification process and corresponding prior probabilities calculated based on the feature set which will make classifier to assign the label cancer to the given article

6.1.2. Decision Tree

Decision tree[14] contains nodes and leaf wherein nodes represent the classifying conditions and leaf represent classifying labels. The labels are selected based on the classifying conditions satisfied at the node stage. The process starts with the input of text input from the root node and the given text input is split into two at the first stage. This process is repeated till the leaf cannot be further split into. The classifying conditions may be made up of presence of absence of words, similarity or dissimilarity of words in the document. The Decision tree also uses Part of Speech tagging to create nodes and leafs.

6.1.3. Support Vector Machine

Support Vector Machine [15] techniques consider the given text input as multidimensional space wherein the input is scattered on the multidimensional space. SVM divide the space into hyperplanes (n-1 sub planes in n dimensional plane) and those hyperplanes are selected which minimize the distances from the words within the planes and but maximises the distance between the planes.

For example let us consider a two dimensional space which contains positives and negatives words. SVM divides the space into hyperplanes (here it is as two disconnected subspace which are separated by a line) and calculates the distance from the hyperplane for each word. Then the task is to select the hyperplane which minimizes the distance for each word from the subspace/line and maximizes the distances between subspaces. Words which are closer to the hyperplane/line form the support vector for that hyperplane or subspace.

6.2 Unsupervised methods[1]

6.2.1 Clustering methods
To group the given input text into clusters so that words in the same cluster are similar and different clusters are dissimilar. The clustering can be done in two ways hierarchical (agglomerative) clustering and partitioning clustering (k-means clustering). In the clustering method Term Frequency-Inverse Document Frequency (IF-DFT) algorithm (weight of a term is proportional to the number of times the term appears in each document) is used to create the clusters

7. Language Modelling [1,16]
Language modelling involves assigning probability to words and sentences. It helps to predict the sequence of words which are likely to be present in a text input. Language models deals with sparse or unknown words through the use of Smoothing algorithm

Zipf's Law[17]
Zipf's Law is an important concept in the language modelling which deals with the words frequency and its weight or rank in a corpus.
When word are ranked by its frequency in a given text input, then frequency * rank of the frequency is equal to a constant
i.e if frequency of word is f and rank of the words frequency is r then
$f*r = c$

7.1. Hidden Markov Models[18]
Hidden Markov Models is defined by a set of states and its associated transition probabilities and output or emission probabilities. Transition probabilities are calculated when the transition happens from state to another state. The states are hidden in the Models but output of each transition is observable with certain probabilities

7.2. n-grams models[19]
An ngram is a continuous sequence of n items in a text where one can predict the nth word from the previous words. 3gram represents continuous sequence of 3 words wherein we can predict the third word from the previous 2 words

8. Information Retrieval and NLP
The starting phase of an automated NLP system involves information retrieval. Some of the information retrieval concepts related to NLP are discussed below

8.1. Latent Semantic Analysis (LSA) and Latent Semantic Indexing (LSI) [20]
In information retrieval process text input is treated as a Document Term matrix wherein rows represents terms, column represents documents. TF_IDF is used to represents the weight of the terms in the text input.

Latent Semantic Analysis (LSA) is used to uncover the meaning of the text in response to the queries during the information retrieval process. LSA uses Singular Value Decomposition techniques to reduce the dimensionality of the Document-Term matrix by grouping the similar words in given text.

9. Software to carry out NLP tasks

The following table gives the list of software available to carry out NLP tasks

Table-2 List of Software

Name of the software	Type	URL
Standford NLP[21]	Open source	www.nlp.stanford.edu
NLTK with python[22]	Open source	www.python.org www.nltk.org
R Statistical Package and R-Studio 1. OpenNLP 2. tm 3. rNLP	Open source	https://www.r-project.org/ https://www.rstudio.com/products/rpackages/

10. Conclusion

This chapter revisited the concepts and methods of Natural Language Processing Systems.

11. References

1. Manning, C. D., & Schütze, H. (1999). *Foundations of statistical natural language processing* (Vol. 999). Cambridge: MIT press.
2. Liddy, E. D. (2001). Natural language processing.
3. Hutchins, W. J. (1986). *Machine translation: past, present, future* (p. 66). Chichester: Ellis Horwood.
4. Spyns, P. (1996). Natural language processing. *Methods of information in medicine*, 35(4), 285-301.

5. Cronin, T. (2014). Automation of Medical Record Risk Factor Tagging Using Machine Learning and Natural Language Processing Methods.
6. Friedman, C., Shagina, L., Lussier, Y., & Hripcsak, G. (2004). Automated encoding of clinical documents based on natural language processing. *Journal of the American Medical Informatics Association, 11*(5), 392-402.
7. Demner-Fushman, D., Chapman, W. W., & McDonald, C. J. (2009). What can natural language processing do for clinical decision support?. Journal of biomedical informatics, 42(5), 760-772.
8. Szlosek, D. A., & Ferrett, J. (2016). Using Machine Learning and Natural Language Processing Algorithms to Automate the Evaluation of Clinical Decision Support in Electronic Medical Record Systems. *eGEMs, 4*(3).
9. Alemzadeh, H., & Devarakonda, M. (2017, February). An NLP-based cognitive system for disease status identification in electronic health records. In *Biomedical & Health Informatics (BHI), 2017 IEEE EMBS International Conference on* (pp. 89-92). IEEE.
10. Zeng, Q. T., Goryachev, S., Weiss, S., Sordo, M., Murphy, S. N., & Lazarus, R. (2006). Extracting principal diagnosis, co-morbidity and smoking status for asthma research: evaluation of a natural language processing system. *BMC medical informatics and decision making, 6*(1), 30.
11. Medhat, W., Hassan, A., & Korashy, H. (2014). Sentiment analysis algorithms and applications: A survey. *Ain Shams Engineering Journal, 5*(4), 1093-1113
12. Collobert, R., Weston, J., Bottou, L., Karlen, M., Kavukcuoglu, K., & Kuksa, P. (2011). Natural language processing (almost) from scratch. *Journal of Machine Learning Research, 12*(Aug), 2493-2537.
13. Go, A., Bhayani, R., & Huang, L. (2009). Twitter sentiment classification using distant supervision. *CS224N Project Report, Stanford, 1*(2009), 12.

14. Brill, E. (1995). Transformation-based error-driven learning and natural language processing: A case study in part-of-speech tagging. *Computational linguistics, 21*(4), 543-565.
15. Collobert, R., & Weston, J. (2008, July). A unified architecture for natural language processing: Deep neural networks with multitask learning. In *Proceedings of the 25th international conference on Machine learning* (pp. 160-167). ACM.
16. Winograd, T. (1972). Understanding natural language. *Cognitive psychology, 3*(1), 1-191.
17. Piantadosi, S. T. (2014). Zipf's word frequency law in natural language: A critical review and future directions. *Psychonomic bulletin & review, 21*(5), 1112-1130.
18. Huang, X. D., Ariki, Y., & Jack, M. A. (1990). *Hidden Markov models for speech recognition* (Vol. 2004). Edinburgh: Edinburgh university press.
19. Brown, P. F., Desouza, P. V., Mercer, R. L., Pietra, V. J. D., & Lai, J. C. (1992). Class-based n-gram models of natural language. *Computational linguistics, 18*(4), 467-479.
20. Landauer, T. K. (2006). *Latent semantic analysis*. John Wiley & Sons, Ltd.
21. Manning, C. D., Surdeanu, M., Bauer, J., Finkel, J. R., Bethard, S., & McClosky, D. (2014, June). The stanford corenlp natural language processing toolkit. In *ACL (System Demonstrations)* (pp. 55-60).
22. Bird, S., Klein, E., & Loper, E. (2009). *Natural language processing with Python: analyzing text with the natural language toolkit*. " O'Reilly Media, Inc.".

Chapter5: Factor analysis revisited – An overview with the help of SPSS, SAS and R packages

Editor, International Journal of Statistics and Medical Informatics

1. Introduction

Numerous research articles and books published on Factor Analysis as it is widely applied in many of the disciplines such as Psychology & behaviour sciences and marketing where more number of observed variables is used. Factor analysis is used to reduce the number of variables which are correlated among themselves by defining them into few factors which are linear combinations of the original variables and it also studies the underlying structure in the data set. Factor analysis [1, 2] is introduced by Spearman a century ago[3, 2,]. This chapter provides an overview of Factor Analysis and how to conduct a Factor Analysis using SAS, SPSS and R statistical packages through a hypothetical data set.

2. Similarity and Dissimilarity between Factor Analysis and Principal Component Analysis (PCA) [5]

Whenever we conduct Factor Analysis, there are questions like whether we can use Factor Analysis or PCA, both methods are same or different will arise. Factor Analysis and PCA have both similarities and dissimilarities among them. Factor Analysis differs from PCA, where components are created from linear combination of original variables. The main aim of PCA is to explain the total variance of the observed variables through the principal components whereas factor analysis aims to study the structure in the dataset. The similarity between both factor analysis and PCA lies in usage of techniques such as extraction, rotation and number of factors or components to be retained in the analysis.

3. Types of Factor Analysis [6]

There are two types of factor analysis one is exploratory factor analysis and another is confirmatory factor analysis. Exploratory factor analysis is used to find out the relationship between the variables under study whereas confirmatory factor analysis is used to test hypothesis about the relationship between component (Factor) structure and original variables under study.

4. Exploratory Factor Analysis[7]

While carrying out the exploratory factor analysis we need to decide about the method of extraction of factors, number of factors to be retained in the dataset, factor rotation method and computing the factor scores method.

The factors can be extracted or determined by using the following methods

a. Method of Principal Component[8,9]

Principal component method is used to extract factors or components from the set of observed variables which are linear combination of the observed variables. Normally the first principal component will represent the highest variance followed by the second and third and so on. Here total number of factors or components will be equal to total number of observed variables. However the number of components to be retained is find out by the using the following methods

Deciding on the number of factors to be retained

i. Kaiser's method- Eigenvalue based[10]

Kaiser uses a technique which decides the number of factors to be retained based on the eigenvalues of the factors which are greater than 1. Eigenvalues are the variance of the principal components or factors. Eigenvalue and Eigenvectors are defined as follows

Eigenvalue and Eigenvectors

If we are having a matrix A of n x n dimension and if the following is true

$$A\lambda = \lambda k \qquad \ldots\ldots(1)$$

Then λ is the Eigenvalue and k is the Eigenvector for eigenvalue λ for the matrix A.

The Eigenvalue and Eigenvector can be found out by solving the following equation

$$|A-\lambda I| \, k = 0 \qquad \ldots\ldots(2)$$

For example if A and I is defined as follows then λ is calculated using

$$A = \begin{pmatrix} 5 & 2 \\ 2 & 5 \end{pmatrix} \qquad I = \begin{pmatrix} 1 & 0 \\ 0 & 1 \end{pmatrix} \qquad \text{then } \lambda \text{ is determined}$$

using

$$A-\lambda I = 0 \qquad \ldots\ldots(3)$$

$$\left| \begin{pmatrix} 5 & 2 \\ 2 & 5 \end{pmatrix} - \begin{pmatrix} \lambda & 0 \\ 0 & \lambda \end{pmatrix} \right| = 0$$

$$\begin{bmatrix} 5-\lambda & 2 \\ 2 & 5-\lambda \end{bmatrix}$$

$(5-\lambda)(5-\lambda) - 2*2 = 0$
$25 - 5\lambda - 5\lambda + \lambda^2 - 4 = 0$
$\lambda^2 - 10\lambda + 21 = 0 \qquad \ldots\ldots(4)$

by solving the equation(4)

We find $\lambda=7$ and $\lambda=3$ and for each λ we need to find the eigenvectors.

We need to find a eigenvector for eigenvalue $\lambda=7$ which satisfy

$$\left(\begin{pmatrix} 5 & 2 \\ 2 & 5 \end{pmatrix} - 7 \times \begin{pmatrix} 1 & 0 \\ 0 & 1 \end{pmatrix}\right) \times \begin{pmatrix} k1 \\ k2 \end{pmatrix} = 0$$

Solving the above equation we get eigenvector = $\begin{pmatrix} -1 \\ -1 \end{pmatrix}$

and similarly for $\lambda=3$, we find eigenvector= $\begin{pmatrix} -1 \\ 1 \end{pmatrix}$

ii. **Cattel's method- Scree plot technique[11]**

Cattel's suggested scree plot technique to decide the number of factors wherein the Eigenvalues are plotted against each factor or component. The normal structure of a scree plot will start with a steep descending curve followed by a flat line at the bottom of the plot. The number of factors retained in the analysis will be where curve in the scree plot starts the flat structure and it will be less than 1.

iii. **Velicer's method[12]**

Velicer suggested the Minimum Average Partial test. It involves computing of average squared off diagonal matrix which is calculated after partial outing the first component, followed by next two principal components and so on till n-1 times where n is the number of variables present in the data. The average squared partial correlation values of each iteration sorted in the ascending order with iteration number. The iteration number which resulted in the minimum average squared partial correlation is selected and the number of components associated with the particular iteration is the number of component to be retained in the analysis

iv. **Horn's Parallel Analysis[13]**
   In Horn parallel analysis method, Eigenvalues are computed from a random dataset with a same number of observations and variables present in the dataset under study. Then the original Eigenvalues from the analysis and the estimated Eigenvalues are plotted against the factors or components. The number of factors to be retained will be decided based on the number of factors before the intersection of the two curves.

b. **Principal factor analysis[14]**
   Principal factor analysis is carried out to find out the minimum number of factors which accounts for common variance of the observed variables

c. **Canonical factor analysis[14]**
   Canonical factor analysis defines the number of factors to be retained based on the sample of cases that best represents the dataset

d. **Alpha factor analysis[14]**
   Alpha factor analysis defines the number of factors to be retained based on the sample of variables that best represents the dataset

e. **Maximum Likelihood Factor Analysis[15]**
   This is method is used when the data is normally distributed and it helps to test the significance of the factor loadings and construct confidence interval for the estimates.

f. **Unweighted Least-Squares Method[16]**
   This method extracts the factors by minimizing the sum of squared deviation between the observed and recalculated correlation matrix using unweighted least square principles.

g. **Generalized Least-Squares Method[17]**
   GKarl G. Jöreskog et.al applied Aitken's Generalized Least Square principle to minimize the sum of squared deviation between the observed and recalculated correlation matrix with help of observed variance-covarince matrix as weight matrix

h. image component analysis
The image component analysis decides the number of factors based on the correlation matrix of predicted variables rather than actual variables where the variables are predicted from the other variables using multiple regression technique.

5. Factor Rotation Methods
Factor rotation methods provide as with an optimum structures of factors in a given data set. The most popular rotation is method is Varimax rotation method

a. Varimax rotation[18]
This methods gives us the smaller of variables which high factor loadings for each factor and this helps us to interpret the component in a clear way

b. Quartimax[19]
This method minimizes the number of factors to represent each variable and this helps to interpret the observed variables in an easy way

c. Equamax[20]
This method combines both Varimax and Quartimax methods and helps us to easily interpret both the variables and the factors

d. Direct Oblimin [21,22]
This is non-orthogonal (oblique) rotation method which helps to get simple structures from the factors

e. Promax[23] – This method is also a non-orthogonal rotation method where the factors are correlated

6. Factor Score Computing Methods [24]
Factor scores represent estimates of common part of the variable. The following methods can be used to compute the factor scores for future analysis purpose

a. Weighted Least Squares
Barlette's weighted least square method can be used to estimate factor scores if multivariate normality assumption is valid. Here original variables are considered as dependent

variable and factors are treated as independent variable and factor scores are the unknown coefficients.
b. Regression method
Regression or exact factor score methods use the estimated parameters from a factor analysis to define linear combinations of observed variables that generate factor scores
c. Anderson Rubin method
This is method ensures that the factors are uncorrelated and estimated scores will be standardized score.

7. Sample Size for Factor Analysis[25]
Number of recommendation by different authors has been suggested as a rule of thumb it starts from 100 to 1000 observations. The sample size should be 5 times as many as the variables and if the variables are highly correlated then lesser number of observations may also be sufficient.

In this example we will use principal component analysis to extract the factors from the hypothetical data set with 10 variables on using SPSS [26], SAS [27] and R[28] codes.

In SPSS, please select the following options
Analyze
    Factor
        Descriptives
            Correlation matrix
                KMO-Bartlet's test of sphercity
        Extraction
            Method
                Principal Component Method
            Analyse
                Correlation matrix
            Extract
                Based on Eigenvalues greater than 1
        Rotation
            Varimax
        Scores
            Regression

SPSS output

Table-1: Sphercity test

KMO and Bartlett's Test		
Kaiser-Meyer-Olkin Measure of Sampling Adequacy.		.834
Bartlett's Test of Sphericity	Approx. Chi-Square	1170.650
	df	36
	Sig.	.000

The above table shows that the KMO score is 0.834 which is above the threshold of 0.6 and as the p value is less than 0.05 we reject the null hypothesis that the variables are orthogonal and factor analysis can be continued

Table-2 : Communalities

Communalities		
	Initial	Extraction
x1	1.000	.758
x2	1.000	.859
x3	1.000	.911
x4	1.000	.724
x5	1.000	.772
x6	1.000	.684
x7	1.000	.641
x8	1.000	.575
x9	1.000	.709
Extraction Method: Principal Component Analysis.		

Here in the above table extraction column gives the calculated variance for each variable accounted by all the principal components (factors). If the extracted communalities are above 0.5 we can retain the particular variable. In the above table all the commonalities are above 0.5, the extracted components are enough to represent the observed variables.

Table-3: Total Variance

Total Variance Explained									
Component	Initial Eigenvalues			Extraction Sums of Squared Loadings			Rotation Sums of Squared Loadings		
	Total	% of Variance	Cumulative %	Total	% of Variance	Cumulative %	Total	% of Variance	Cumulative %
1	4.361	48.457	48.457	4.361	48.457	48.457	4.312	47.916	47.916
2	1.202	13.359	61.816	1.202	13.359	61.816	1.197	13.304	61.220
3	1.069	11.878	73.695	1.069	11.878	73.695	1.123	12.475	73.695
4	.829	9.215	82.910						
5	.787	8.743	91.652						
6	.319	3.550	95.202						
7	.229	2.542	97.743						
8	.134	1.483	99.227						
9	.070	.773	100.000						
Extraction Method: Principal Component Analysis.									

In the above table-3, initial Eigenvalues are shown given with three columns, **total,% of variance and cumulative variance**.
- When we add the **total column** it will be equal to the number of variables and number of components(factors) under study i.e 9 and
- **% of variance column** gives overall percentage explained each component (factor)

- **cumulative column** gives the cumulative percentage explained by retained components as in the example only three components retained based on the criteria (Eigenvalues should be greater than 1 to be retained) and cumulative variance explained by the retained components(factor) are 74% and 26% of information is last and we can continue with the factor analysis
- Extraction sum of squared loadings and rotation sum of squared loadings provide the factor loadings for each retained components

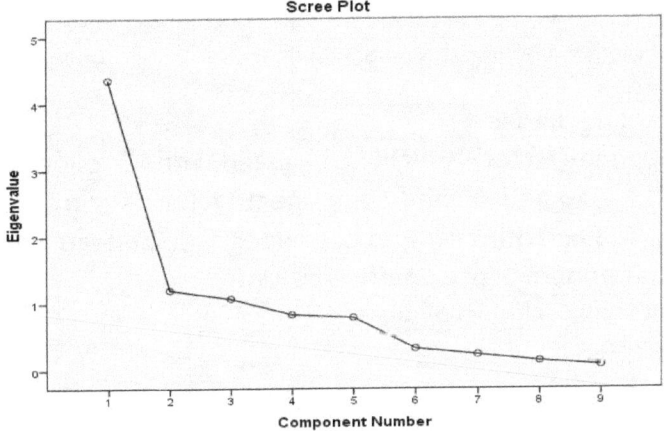

The above scree plot also displays only three factors which are having Eigenvalues more than 1 and the curve starts as a flat line in the bottom after the step drop

Table-4: Component Matrix

Component Matrix[a]			
	Component		
	1	2	3
x1	.815	.048	-.301
x2	.885	.105	-.253
x3	.943	.051	-.136
x4	.843	-.055	.101
x5	.858	-.097	.161
x6	.740	-.175	.324
x7	-.026	.749	-.284
x8	-.090	-.725	-.203
x9	.137	.240	.795

Extraction Method: Principal Component Analysis.
a. 3 components extracted.

First component(factor) is highly correlated with x3 followed by x1, x2, x3, x4, x5, x6 and second component(factor) is correlated with x7 followed x8 and third component(factor) is correlated with x9.

Table-5 Component Score Coefficient Matrix

Component Score Coefficient Matrix			
	Component		
	1	2	3
x1	.218	.095	-.244
x2	.227	.133	-.189
x3	.228	.068	-.089
x4	.182	-.062	.107
x5	.180	-.107	.155
x6	.137	-.201	.288
x7	.007	.662	-.138
x8	.020	-.554	-.304
x9	-.063	.050	.767

Extraction Method: Principal Component Analysis.
Rotation Method: Varimax with Kaiser Normalization.
Component Scores.

Component scores are stored for each observation which can be used for further analysis with 3 principal component or factors

SAS Code and Output

proc factor data = mydata method=prin priors=one mineigen=1 rotate=varimax round;

var x1 x2 x3 x4 x5 x6 x7 x8 x9;
run;
Section1- Prior Communality Estimates: ONE

Eigenvalues of the Correlation Matrix: Total = 9 Average = 1

		Eigenvalue	Difference	Proportion	Cumulative
	1	4.36110702	3.15876321	0.4846	0.4846
	2	1.20234381	0.13328105	0.1336	0.6182
	3	1.06906277	0.23970892	0.1188	0.7369
	4	0.82935385	0.04250567	0.0922	0.8291
	5	0.78684818	0.46739146	0.0874	0.9165
	6	0.31945672	0.09071709	0.0355	0.9520
	7	0.22873963	0.09523420	0.0254	0.9774
	8	0.13350543	0.06392283	0.0148	0.9923
	9	0.06958260		0.0077	1.0000

3 factors will be retained by the MINEIGEN criterion.

Section-2 : Factor Pattern

	Factor1	Factor2	Factor3
x1	82 *	5	-30
x2	89 *	10	-25

x3	94 *	5	-14
x4	84 *	-5	10
x5	86 *	-10	16
x6	74 *	-17	32
x7	-3	75 *	-28
x8	-9	-72 *	-20
x9	14	24	80 *

Printed values are multiplied by 100 and rounded to the nearest integer. Values greater than 0.49563 are flagged by an

Section-3: Final Communality Estimates: Total = 6.632514

x1	x2	x3	x4	x5
x6	x7	x8	x9	

0.75752517   0.85916423   0.91063578   0.72428786
0.77181082 0.68373085 0.64146989 0.57470328 0.70918573

The above SAS program provides

- Section-1: Same number of Components (factors) i.e 3 to be retained in the analysis as of SPSS and The total variance explained is also close to 74%
- Section-2: First component(factor) correlated with x3 followed by x1, x2, x3, x4, x5, x6 and second component(factor) is correlated with x7 followed x8 and third component(factor) is correlated with x9.
- Section-3: Here all the final communality estimates are above 0.5 and close to the initial communality 1

R Code and output
>analysis <- princomp (mydata, cor=TRUE)
>summary (analysis)
>loadings (analysis)
>plot (analysis)

Output
Section: summary (analysis)
Importance of components:

	Comp.1	Comp.2	Comp.3	Comp.4	Comp.5	Comp.6	Comp.7	Comp.8
Standard deviation	2.0836402	1.0973268	1.0348153	0.91133318	0.88307147	0.56582678	0.49496388	0.36920225
Proportion of Variance	0.4823952	0.1337918	0.1189825	0.09228091	0.08664614	0.03557333	0.02722103	0.01514559
Cumulative Proportion	0.4823952	0.6161870	0.7351695	0.82745039	0.91409652	0.94966985	0.97689088	0.99203647

Section: Loadings:

```
   Comp.1 Comp.2 Comp.3 Comp.4 Comp.5 Comp.6 Comp.7 Comp.8 Comp.9
X1 -0.374        -0.211  0.514  0.179         0.556  0.246  0.382
X2 -0.392        -0.195  0.377  0.110 -0.108 -0.315 -0.721 -0.142
X3 -0.415        -0.108  0.127        -0.645  0.607
X4 -0.399               -0.271 -0.733 -0.400  0.237 -0.101
X5 -0.402         0.110 -0.267  0.803        -0.139  0.286
X6 -0.358         0.270 -0.498  0.610 -0.380         0.168
X7  0.188 -0.564 -0.504 -0.257        -0.111 -0.159         0.531
X8  0.205  0.725        -0.124 -0.123 -0.263 -0.105  0.558
X9        -0.380  0.749  0.334 -0.112        -0.156         0.357
```

Section: plot(analysis)

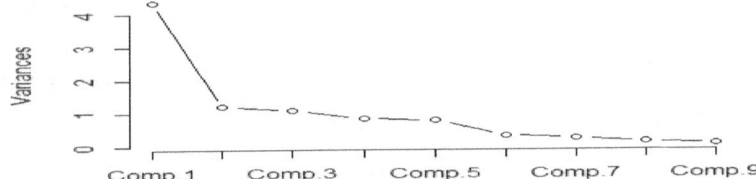

The above R program provides

- Section-1: Same number of Components (factors) i.e 3 to be retained in the analysis as of SPSS and The total variance explained is also close to 74%
- Section-2: First component(factor) correlated with x3 followed by x1, x2, x3, x4, x5, x6 and second component(factor) is correlated with x7 followed x8 and third component(factor) is correlated with x9.

Conclusion

This chapter revisited the concepts and methods of factor analysis using SPSS, SAS and R software

References

1. Holzinger, K. J., & Harman, H. H. (1941). Factor analysis; a synthesis of factorial methods.
2. Cartel, R. B. (1965). Factor analysis: An introduction to essential I. The purpose of underlying models. *Biometrics, 21*(1), 190-235.
3. Pearson, Karl. "Principal components analysis." *The London, Edinburgh and Dublin Philosophical Magazine and Journal* 6.2 (1901): 566.
4. Kane, H., & Brand, C. (1905). The importance of Spearman's g. *The occidental quarterly, 3*(1), 7-30.
5. Joliffe, I. T., & Morgan, B. J. T. (1992). Principal component analysis and exploratory factor analysis. *Statistical methods in medical research, 1*(1), 69-95.
6. Thompson, B. (2004). Exploratory and confirmatory factor analysis: Understanding concepts and applications. American Psychological Association.
7. Fabrigar, L. R., & Wegener, D. T. (2011). Exploratory factor analysis. Oxford University Press.
8. https://www.ibm.com/support/knowledgecenter/en/SSLVMB_23.0.0/spss/base/idh_fact_rot.html
9. Lawley, D. N., & Maxwell, A. E. (1971). Factor analysis as a statistical method (Vol. 18). London: Butterworths.
10. Kaiser, H. F. (1960). The application of electronic computers to factor analysis. *Educational and psychological measurement, 20*(1), 141-151.
11. Cattell, R. B. (1966). The scree test for the number of factors. *Multivariate behavioral research, 1*(2), 245-276.
12. Velicer, W. F. (1976). Determining the number of components from the matrix of partial correlations. *Psychometrika, 41*(3), 321-327.

13. Horn, J. L. (1965). A rationale and test for the number of factors in factor analysis. *Psychometrika, 30*(2), 179-185.
14. McDonald, R. P. (1970). The theoretical foundations of principal factor analysis, canonical factor analysis, and alpha factor analysis. *British Journal of Mathematical and Statistical Psychology, 23*(1), 1-21.
15. Jöreskog, K. G. (1967). A general approach to confirmatory maximum likelihood factor analysis. ETS Research Report Series, 1967(2), 183-202.
16. Jöreskog, K. G., & Sörbom, D. (1986). LISREL VI: Analysis of linear structural relationships by maximum likelihood, instrumental variables, and least squares methods. Scientific Software.
17. Jöreskog, K. G., & Goldberger, A. S. (1972). Factor analysis by generalized least squares. *Psychometrika, 37*(3), 243-260.
18. Kaiser, H. F. (1958). The varimax criterion for analytic rotation in factor analysis. *Psychometrika, 23*(3), 187-200.
19. Neuhaus, J. O., & Wrigley, C. (1954). The quartimax method. *British Journal of Statistical Psychology, 7*(2), 81-91.
20. Kaiser, H. F. (1974). A note on the equamax criterion. *Multivariate behavioral research, 9*(4), 501-503.
21. Jennrich, R. I. (1979). Admissible values of γ in direct oblimin rotation. *Psychometrika, 44*(2), 173-177.
22. Jennrich, R. I., & Sampson, P. F. (1966). Rotation for simple loadings. *Psychometrika, 31*(3), 313-323.
23. Hendrickson, A. E., & White, P. O. (1964). Promax: A quick method for rotation to oblique simple structure. *British journal of statistical psychology, 17*(1), 65-70.
24. Costello, A. B. (2009). Getting the most from your analysis. *Pan, 12*(2), 131-146.
25. Mundfrom, D. J., Shaw, D. G., & Ke, T. L. (2005). Minimum sample size recommendations for conducting factor analyses. *International Journal of Testing, 5*(2), 159-168.
26. SPSS Inc. Released 2008. SPSS Statistics for Windows, Version 17.0. Chicago: SPSS Inc.

27. SAS and all other SAS Institute Inc. product or service names are registered trademarks or trademarks of SAS Institute Inc. in the USA and other countries. ® indicates USA registration.
28. Team, R. C. (2014). R: A language and environment for statistical computing. R Foundation for Statistical Computing, Vienna, Austria. 2013.

Chapter6: Post-hoc and multiple comparison test – An overview with SAS and R Statistical Package

Editor, International Journal of Statistics and Medical Informatics (ISJMI)

1. Introduction

When a researcher wants to test the difference between three or more drug's effect on controlling serum cholesterol, one way Analysis of Variance (ANOVA) method can be used to find out whether mean cholesterol level between the groups are statistically different or not. If there is a difference between the drug's effects found on controlling the serum cholesterol then Post-hoc and multiple comparison tests [1, 2, 3] can used to find out which pair of drugs differ from each other.

Normally a student t-test or equivalent non parametric test such as Mann Whitney U test can be used to test whether the two means differ or not. The problem with the t-test or its non-parametric equivalent tests is that it increases the overall Type I error or family wise error rate.

2. Type I error and Family Wise Error Rate (FWER)

The type 1 error for single test (error wrongly rejecting the null hypothesis when it is actually true) is denoted by α.

Table: 1 – Type I and Type II error

Decision from the Test	Null Hypothesis True Status : True	Null Hypothesis True Status : False
Decision from the test : Reject Null Hypothesis based on the sample data	False Positive (α-Type I error)	True Positive (1- α)

Decision from the test : Accept Null Hypothesis based on the sample data	True Negative $(1-\beta)$	False Negative (β- Type II error)

If n multiple tests are carried out then the cumulative or Family Wise Error Rate is calculated as below

$\alpha_n = 1 - (1 - \alpha_i)^n$ where n is the number of comparison being tested and i is the ith comparison

Post Hoc and Multiple Comparison Tests

Post Hoc tests are used to compare the pair of treatment means while controlling the Family Wise Error Rate. These tests are conducted normally after the one way ANOVA [4, 5] returns significant results.

The following sections discusses various multiple comparison tests [6] available with its usefulness and limitations

1. **Bonferroni-adjusted multiple t-tests(Dunn) [1,2]**
   Bonferroni adjusted multiple t-tests (Dunn) is easy to compute and flexible to use for any multiple comparison while controlling the FWER. It does not require an ANOVA to be significant as it falls under planned comparison procedure.
   Positives
   a. It is easy to compute
   b. It controls the FWER
   c. It does not require ANOVA to be significant
   Limitations
   a. Its lacks power due to the fact that it assumes null hypothesis is true for all the tests in consideration

2. **Sidak test** [1,2]
   Sidak test is having slightly higher power than Bonferroni test while retaining the FWER
   Positives
   a. It is easy to compute
   b. It controls the FWER
   c. Slightly powerful than Bonferroni
   Limitations
   a. Lacks power
3. **Dunnett's test**[1,2]
   Dunnett's test tests only compare the control group with the other groups. . In each pair wise comparisons control group will be present. It does not compare the other groups with each other
   Positives
   a. It is exact procedure to compare a control with the other groups in consideration
   Limitations
   a. Limited application due to the fact that it is useful when one compares the control with the other groups
   b. Equal variance assumption to be met
4. **Tukey honestly significant difference (HSD) test** [8]
   Tukey's test works on the Studentized range statistic called Q statistics which calculates the critical value based on the number of groups and number of sample observation in the group. Tukey's test assumes the sample observations being tested are independent within and between the groups, group means are normally distributed and assumes equal variance among the group.
   Positives
   a. It maintains the alpha level at the desired range when the three assumptions are met
   b. It is useful when sample sizes are not equal among groups and
   c. All pairwise comparisons are carried out

Limitations
a. Powerful
b. It assumes equal variances for the groups which may not be the case always

5. **Games and Howell's modification of Tukey's HSD** [9]
It is modification of Tukey's HSD test and used when the unequal variance assumption is violated
Positives
a. It is useful when unequal variances assumption is violated while using the Tukey's HSD test
Limitations
a. It is less conservative when the sample sizes of the groups are small.

6. **Tukey's wholly significant difference (WSD) test** [1,2]
It is modification of Tukey's HSD test and used when the unequal variance assumption is violated
Positives
a. It is useful when unequal variances assumption is violated while using the Tukey's HSD test
Limitations
a. It is less conservative when the sample sizes of the groups are small.

7. **Newman-Keuls test(Student-Newman-Keuls- SNK)** [10]
It is one of the step down procedure where in the difference between the largest and smallest means are compared first if it is significant continue the next set of pairs (second largest vs smallest or second smallest vs largest) or stop if the pair is not significant. This test is continued till a non-significant pair comparison is reached
Positives
a. This test is useful when the number of pairwise comparisons are more
b. Liberal than Dunn's Test
Limitations
a. FWER is not controlled

8. **Ryan Einot Gabriel Welch q test (REGWQ)** [1,11]
   It is one of the step down procedure wherein the difference between the largest and smallest means are compared first if it is significant continue the next set of pairs (second largest vs smallest or second smallest vs largest) or stop if the pair is not significant. This test is continued till a non-significant pair comparison is reached
   Positives
   a. FWER is controlled
   b. Liberal and powerful than Tukey's Test
   Limitations
   a. Not useful when the sample size between the groups are different
   b. Less powerful than REGWF test

9. **Ryan Einot Gabriel Welch F test (REGWF))** [1,11]
   This test is based on F statistic rather than the q statistic
   Positives
   a. FWER is controlled
   b. Powerful than REGWQ test
   Limitations
   a. Not useful when the sample size between the groups are different

10. **The Shaffer-Ryan test)** [1,11]
    It is a modified version of REGWF test which
    Positives
    c. FWER is controlled
    d. Powerful than REGWQ and REGWF test
    Limitations
    b. Not useful when the sample size between the groups are different

11. **The Least Significant Difference test (LSD)/ Fisher's LSD** [12]
    It is the simplest of the entire multiple comparison test and it controls the FWER only when 3 means are tested.
    Positives
    a. Most Powerful test
    Limitations

a. Very poor in controlling the FWER

12. The Fisher-Hayter test [13]

It is a modification of Fishers LSD test

Positives
a. Easy to use
b. Controls the FWER

Limitations
a. Useful only for pairwise contrasts
b. Less Powerful when number of comparisons are less

13. Waller-Duncan test [1,2]

It is different from the other multiple comparison tests as it uses Bayesian approach wherein it minimizes the overall loss function which is a sum of loss functions for all comparisons

14. Dunnett's T3 [1,2]

This test is used to test the pairwise comparison, groups are having unequal variance and group sample size is small.

Positives
a. Controls FWER
b. It is useful when variances of the groups are unequal
c. It is useful when the sample size is small

Limitations
a. FWER may exceed the desired level when the variances are equal

15. Tamhane' T2 [1,2,14]

This test is used to test the pairwise comparison and groups are having unequal variance

Positives
a. Controls FWER
b. It is useful when variances of the groups are unequal

Limitations
a. FWER may exceed the desired level when the variances are equal

16. **Howell and Dunnett's C** [1,2]
    This test is used to test the pairwise comparison groups which are having unequal variance. This test is useful when the sample size is large
    Positives
    a. Controls FWER
    b. It is useful when variances of the groups are unequal
    c. It is useful when the sample size is large
    Limitations
    b. FWER may exceed the desired level when the variances are equal
17. **The Tukey-Kramer test** [13]
    It is a modified version of Tukey's test when the groups are having unequal sample size
    Positives
    a. When the sample size is unequal
    Limitations
    a. Useful only when fixed number of comparisons are used
18. **The Miller-Winer test** [1,2]
    This test is used when the sample size of the groups are unequal.
    Positives
    a. When the sample size is unequal
19. **Hochberg's GT2 test** [1,2]
    This test is used when the sample size of the groups are unequal.
    Positives
    a. When the sample size is unequal
20. **Gabriel test** [15]
    This test is used when the sample size of the groups are unequal.
    Positives
    b. When the sample size is unequal
21. **The Scheffe test** [16]
    Scheffe test is a flexible and conservative test and is useful for both simple and complex comparisons.

Positives
   a. Controls FWER
   b. Useful when more number of comparison to be used
   c. Useful for both equal and unequal sample sizes
Limitations
   a. It has less power

22. **The Duncan's Multiple Range test** [17]
    It is a modified version of Student Newman Keuls method
    Positives
    d. It is powerful
    Limitations
    b. It does not control the FWER

3.   **Example using SAS® software [7]**
data cholestral;
input treatmentgroup serumcholestrol;
datalines;
2 253
2 253
2 324
2 303
2 247
3 331
2 332
1 319
3 202
2 211
4 230
3 202
3 216
4 220
3 305
3 223
2 229
3 213
3 292

3 211
3 293
1 330
2 264
1 239
4 295
4 277
3 292
2 269
4 338
1 299
3 246
3 273
1 245
3 313
2 309
3 212
3 240
2 207
1 291
3 302
2 211
2 273
3 334
4 269
1 234
4 217
4 336
2 253
3 207
3 228
4 252
2 293
4 257
1 240
2 307

3 280
2 294
3 337
4 350
4 274
4 302
4 283
4 320
3 288
4 212
1 248
4 236
4 340
3 310
2 279
2 310
4 331
1 288
3 222
2 300
2 206
1 204
2 268
2 237
2 226
3 308
;
proc glm;
class **treatmentgroup;**
model **serumcholestrol = treatmentgroup;**
means **treatmentgroup/Lsd** tukey bon Duncan Dunnett Gabriel regwq scheffe sidak waller;
run;

4. Example using R Statistical Package Code

```
>treatmentgroup<-
c(3,1,3,4,2,1,4,1,4,3,2,1,3,1,4,4,3,2,2,1,3,4,1,1,4,2,4,3,1,2,1,2,3,4,4,2
,1,1,4,3,1,2,4,1,3,2,3,1,2,3,1,4,1,2,3,2,2,3,3,4,2,4,4,3,4,4,1,2,1,4,2,3,
3,3,2,4,2,1,1,3,3)
>serumcholestrol<-
c(245,198,122,308,261,282,221,191,191,209,282,274,285,193,265,
273,229,207,257,375,273,269,204,204,229,281,289,309,290,270,21
7,190,286,241,264,234,221,200,227,259,226,237,264,218,255,2622
8,320,247,230,251,386,383,322,369,203,213,222,283,227,260,232,
209,272,213,244,224,287,231,230,290,269,237,257,295,429,225,26
2,224,235,287,293)
>tapply(serumcholestrol, treatmentgroup, mean)
pairwise.t.test(serumcholestrol, treatmentgroup, p.adj = "none")
pairwise.t.test(serumcholestrol, treatmentgroup, p.adj = "bonferroni")
pairwise.t.test(serumcholestrol, treatmentgroup, p.adj = "holm")
pairwise.t.test(serumcholestrol, treatmentgroup, p.adj = "hochberg")
pairwise.t.test(serumcholestrol, treatmentgroup, p.adj = "hommel")
pairwise.t.test(serumcholestrol, treatmentgroup, p.adj = "BH")
pairwise.t.test(serumcholestrol, treatmentgroup, p.adj = "fdr")
pairwise.t.test(serumcholestrol, treatmentgroup, p.adj = "BY")
```

5. Conclusion

This chapter discussed the various post hoc multiple comparison tests, its usefulness and limitation and also provided the SAS and R statistical package codes with the example dataset

References

[1]. Toothaker, L. E. (1993). Multiple comparison procedures (No. 89). Sage.

[2]. Saville, D. J. (1990). Multiple comparison procedures: the practical solution. *The American Statistician, 44*(2), 174-180.

[3]. Kim, H. Y. (2015). Statistical notes for clinical researchers: post-hoc multiple comparisons. Restorative dentistry & endodontics, 40(2), 172-176.

[4]. Ruxton, G. D., & Beauchamp, G. (2008). Time for some a priori thinking about post hoc testing. Behavioral Ecology, 19(3), 690-693.

[5]. Cabral, H. J. (2008). Multiple comparisons procedures. Circulation, 117(5), 698-701.

[6]. Brown, A. M. (2005). A new software for carrying out one-way ANOVA post hoc tests. Computer methods and programs in biomedicine, 79(1), 89-95.

[7]. http:// www.vinaitheerthan.com/posthoctests.php

[8]. Abdi, H., & Williams, L. J. (2010). Tukey's honestly significant difference (HSD) test. Encyclopedia of Research Design. Thousand Oaks, CA: Sage, 1-5.

[9]. Games, P. A., & Howell, J. F. (1976). Pairwise multiple comparison procedures with unequal n's and/or variances: a Monte Carlo study. Journal of Educational and Behavioral Statistics, 1(2), 113-125.

[10]. Abdi, H., & Williams, L. J. (2010). Newman-Keuls test and Tukey test. Encyclopedia of Research Design. Thousand Oaks, CA: Sage, 1-11.

[11]. Ryan, T. H. (1960). Significance tests for multiple comparisons of proportions, variances, and other statistics. Psychological bulletin, 57(4), 318.

[12]. Williams, L. J., & Abdi, H. (2010). Fisher's least significant difference (LSD) test. Encyclopedia of research design, 1-5.

[13]. Richter, S. J., & McCann, M. H. (2012). Using the Tukey–Kramer omnibus test in the Hayter–Fisher procedure. *British Journal of Mathematical and Statistical Psychology, 65*(3), 499-510.

[14]. Tamhane, A. C. (1979). A comparison of procedures for multiple comparisons of means with unequal variances. *Journal of the American Statistical Association*, *74*(366a), 471-480.

[15]. Gabriel, K. R. (1969). Simultaneous test procedures--some theory of multiple comparisons. *The Annals of Mathematical Statistics*, 224-250.

[16]. Scheffe, H. (1999). *The analysis of variance* (Vol. 72). John Wiley & Sons.

[17]. Duncan, D. B. (1955). Multiple range and multiple F tests. *Biometrics*, *11*(1), 1-42.

SAS and all other SAS Institute Inc. product or service names are registered trademarks or trademarks of SAS Institute Inc. in the USA and other countries. ® indicates USA registration.

Chapter7: Application of Quantile regression in clinical research: An overview with the help of R and SAS statistical package

Editor, International Journal of Statistics and Medical Informatics (ISJMI)

1. Introduction

Normally the relationship between two variables x and y is studied using the linear regression equation. Linear regression equation requires normality and homoscedasticity (equal variance) assumptions. When the normality and homoscedasticity assumptions are violated, linear regression estimates are not valid. Quantile regression method overcomes the drawbacks of linear regression and can be applied when the data is skewed and equal variance assumptions are violated. This chapter provides an overview of application of quantile regression in clinical research using R and SAS statistical package.

Linear regression [1] is used to study the relationship between a dependent variable (response variable) and a set of independent variables (predictors). Linear regression provides the average (mean) value of a dependent variable for the specified values of the independent variables. Linear regression is useful when the data is normal and equal variance is assumed. If the data is having outliers and the distribution is skewed either outliers needs to be removed or data to be transformed to make it normal. Sometimes the removal of outliers is not possible as we may lose important information in the data. Hence an alternative methodology which can handle outliers needs to be adopted. Quantile regression [2, 3,4] is one such methodology which can overcome the problem of outliers. Quantile regression estimates quantiles (percentiles) of the dependent variable based on the quantiles (percentiles) of the independent variables. The quantile regression is used in different fields where the data is skewed such as finance and economics [2, 3], environmental science and clinical research.

The following table-1 provides the difference between linear and quantile regression method [5]

Table-1: Linear Regression vs. Quantile Regression

Linear Regression	Quantile Regression
Uses mean in estimating the response variable	Uses quantiles in estimating the response variable
Affected by outliers	Not affected by outliers
Equal variance assumption is needed	Equal variance assumption not necessary
Assumes normality	Distribution free

1. **Quantile regression methodology**

Quantile regression function [2] is defined as follows
For the pth percentile the dependent variable y is defined as
   i. $Q_p(Y) = \inf(y : F(y) \geq p)$ where p is the quantile (0.25, 0.5 and 0.75)

Conditional quantile function of y given x is
   ii. $Q_p(Y/X=x) = \inf(y : F(y/x) \geq p)$

The quantile regression equation is given by
   iii. $Q_p(Y/x) = x^p b(p). 0 < p < 1$

Where b(p) is the quantile coefficient for the quantile values p
In quantile regression the absolute error function will be minimized to obtain the quantile regression coefficients b(p) and it can be done through linear programming methodology
   iv. $\min \sum (|y_i - x^p b|)$

2. **Examples of application of Quantile regression in clinical research[6,7]**
   a. Quantile regression to estimate probabilities of Low birth weight

   When we carry out the analysis to find out the probability of mothers having low birth weight babies, linear regression model based on the average birth weight as a function of different predictors will leave the lower birth weight categories which is not correct as it losses the important

information due to the skewness in the distribution. Quantile regression will be useful in these scenarios as it includes both the lower, middle and upper quantiles in predicting the probabilities of lower birth weight

The following example uses the dataset set from Hosmer book [8] and models the child birth weight based on the mother's weight. SAS Procedure quantreg [9] is used to carried out the quantile regression analysis

SAS Code

proc quantreg data=lbw;
model bwt = lwt/quantile = 0.05 to 0.95 by 0.05
plot=quantplot;

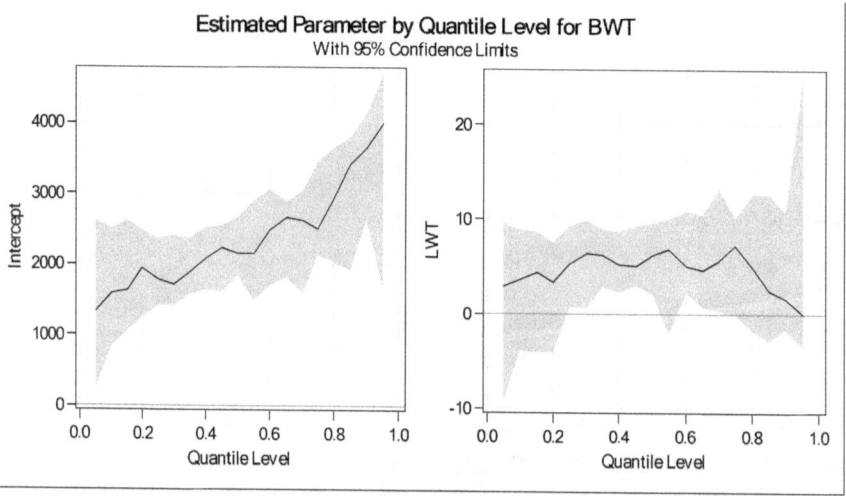

Figure-1: Quantile level of child birth weight with respect to mother's weight

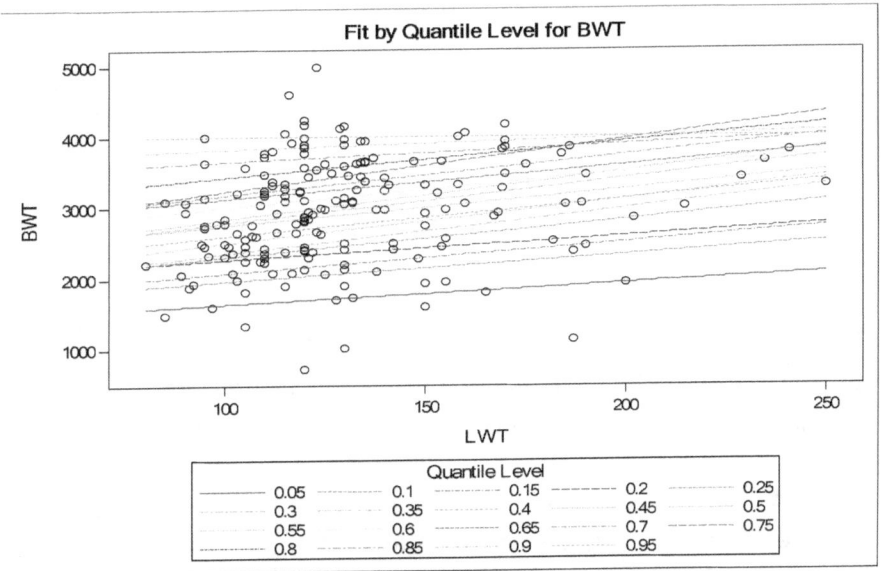

Figure-2: Fit by quantile level of child birth weight with respect to mothers weight

The results provided the information related to different quantiles which clearly shows the effect of mother's weight on the child birth weight and it captures the information related to extreme values which is not captured by the linear regression as shown below in figure-3 (Child birth weight with respect to mothers weight using Linear regression model)

Linear Regression using SAS
    proc reg data=lbw;
    model bwt =lwt

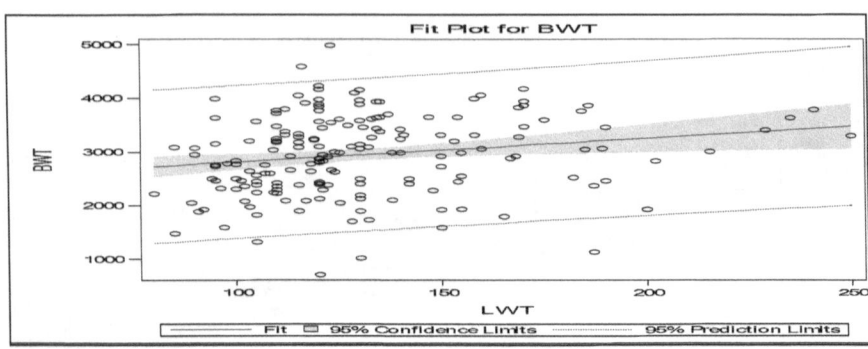

Figure-3 : Fit for child birth weight with respect to mothers weight
Low birth weight example using R statistical package[10]:

The above mentioend low birth weight dataset is used for carrying out the quantile regression and linear regerssion through R statistical package quantreg[11].

library(quantreg)
library(xlsx)
data1 <- read.xlsx("new.xlsx",1,header=T)
summary(data1$LWT)
lw<- rq(data1$BWT~data1$LWT,tau=seq(0.2, 0.8, by=0.1))
lw1<- lm(data1$BWT~data1$LWT)
summary(lw)
summary(lw1)
plot(lw)
plot(lw1)

The following figure shows relationssship between the birth weight of babies and mother weight with respect to quantiles ranging from 0.05 to 0.95 using quantile regression

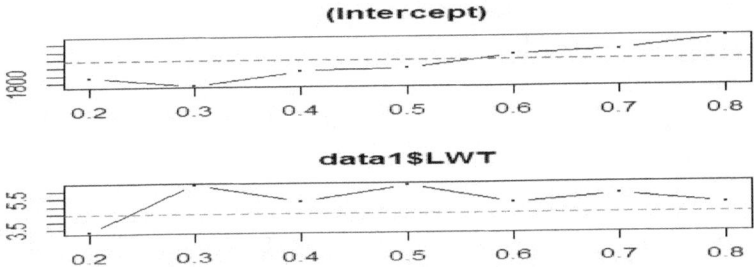

Figure-4: Figure-3 : Fit for child birth weight with respect to mothers weight

The following figure-5 shows relationsship between residual vs fitted values with respect to the birth weight of babies and mother weight using linear regression which is affected by the extreme values especially the lower birth weight

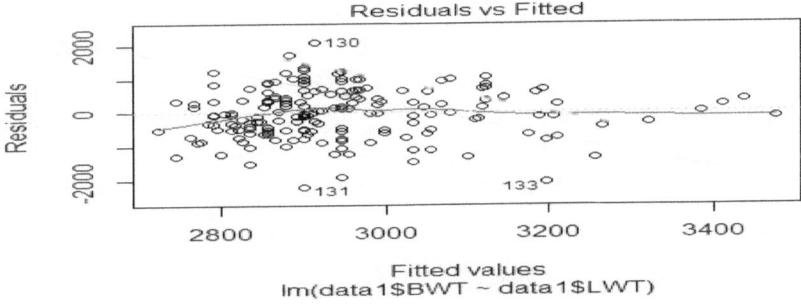

Hence from the above results it can concluded that the quantile regression is capable of handling the extreme values than the linear regression

b. Analysis of health care expenditures

Quantile regression is used to analyse the relationship between health care expending [12, 6] and other variables such as race, ethnicity, gender and other economic factors as normally income and expenditure data distributions are skewed and normal regression estimates may be affected by outliers.

- **Quantile regression in survival analysis**
  Quantile regression can be used to obtain the quantile (percentile) estimates of the survival curve and assess the effects of covariates on the survival rate [13, 14, 15]. When the survival function is given as
  $S(x) = 1- F(x) = 1-p$
  Where $F(x) = F(X<=x) = p$, x is the time to event variable
  Then Quantile estimate Q(p) is given by
  $Q(p) = F^{-1} = x$

3. Conclusion

This chapter provided an overview of quantile regression in the clinical research filed using SAS and R statistical package and also discussed the difference between the quantile regression and the linear regression methods.

References

1. Seber, George AF, and Alan J. Lee. *Linear regression analysis.* Vol. 936. John Wiley & Sons, 2012.
2. Koenker, R. (2005). *Quantile regression* (No. 38). Cambridge university press.
3. Koenker, R. (2017). Quantile Regression: 40 Years On. *Annual Review of Economics, 9*(1).
4. Yu, K., Lu, Z., & Stander, J. (2003). Quantile regression: applications and current research areas. *Journal of the Royal Statistical Society: Series D (The Statistician), 52*(3), 331-350.
5. Beyerlein, A. (2014). Quantile regression—opportunities and challenges from a user's perspective. *American journal of epidemiology, 180*(3), 330-331.
6. Cook, B., & Manning, W. G. (2013). Thinking beyond the mean: a practical guide for using quantile regression methods for health services research. *Shanghai archives of psychiatry, 25*(1), 55.
7. Austin, P. C., Tu, J. V., Daly, P. A., & Alter, D. A. (2005). The use of quantile regression in health care research: a case study examining gender differences in the timeliness of thrombolytic therapy. *Statistics in medicine, 24*(5), 791-816.

8. Hosmer, D.W., Lemeshow, S. and Sturdivant, R.X. (2013) Applied Logistic Regression: Third Edition.
9. https://support.sas.com/documentation/cdl/en/statug/63033/HTML/default/viewer.htm#statug_qreg_sect008.htm (Accessed on 25-Mar-2017)
10. https://cran.r-project.org/web/packages/quantreg/index.html (Accessed on 25-Mar-2017)
11. KOENKER, R. QUANTILE REGRESSION IN R: A VIGNETTE.
12. Chen, J., Vargas-Bustamante, A., Mortensen, K., & Thomas, S. B. (2014). Using quantile regression to examine health care expenditures during the great recession. *Health services research*, *49*(2), 705-730.
13. Peng, L., & Huang, Y. (2008). Survival analysis with quantile regression models. *Journal of the American Statistical Association*, *103*(482), 637-649
14. Yin, G., & Cai, J. (2005). Quantile regression models with multivariate failure time data. *Biometrics*, *61*(1), 151-161.
15. Lin, G., & Rodriguez, R. N. (2013). Using the QUANTLIFE Procedure for Survival Analysis. In *Proceedings of the SAS Global Forum 2013 Conference, Cary, NC: SAS Institute Inc.* Available at http:/support. sas. com/resources/papers/proceedings11/421-2013. pdf.

SAS and all other SAS Institute Inc. product or service names are registered trademarks or trademarks of SAS Institute Inc. in the USA and other countries. ® indicates USA registration.